YOGA OF YARN

A Knitter's Handbook for Self-Discovery

LIZA LAIRD

Foreword by Melanie Falick

Notice

This book is a reference text only, not a medical manual. If you have any medical concerns or conditions consult your doctor before attempting any of the practices in this book.

ISBN: 978-1-7375021-0-4

Copyright © 2022 by Liza Laird

Published in 2022 by RK Press. All rights reserved. No portion of this book may be reproduced, stored in a retrieval system, or transmitted in any form or by any means, mechanical, electronic, photocopying, recording, or otherwise, without written permission from the publisher.

Editor: Melanie Falick
Book Designer: Laura McFadden
Illustrator: Aly Miller
Knitting/Technical Editor: Sue McCain
Copy Editor: Mary Neal Meador

Printed in China
10 9 8 7 6 5 4 3 2 1

The knitter within me honors the knitter within you.

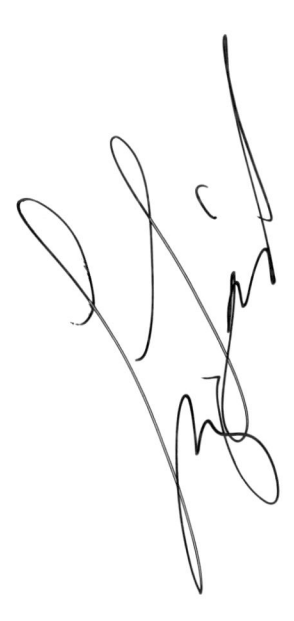

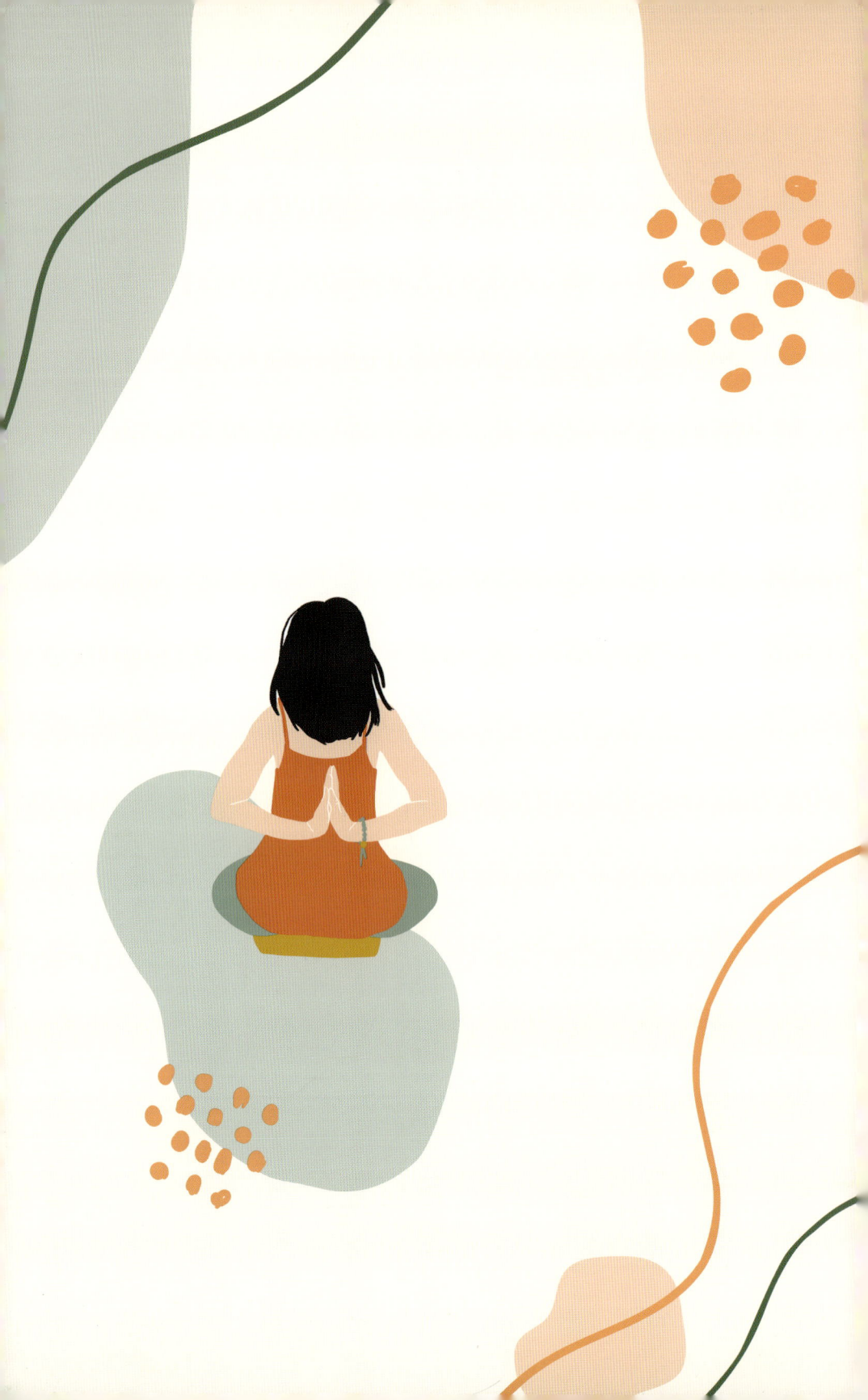

Contents

FOREWORD — viii
INTRODUCTION — x

How to Use This Book — xiv
Six Categories of Explorations — xv
Rest-and-Digest — xvi

Developing a Home Practice — xviii
Sacred Space — xix
Five Minutes to Start — xx

PART 1: BEGINNINGS — 1

Namaste — 2
Power of the Universe — 3
Beginner's Mind — 4
Setting an Intention — 6
Finding Ease — 8
The Art of Sitting — 10
Floor Sitting — 12
Starting with a Strong Foundation — 14
Flow — 18

Meditation — 20
Mantra — 21
Mindfulness — 22
Knitter's Mudras — 24
Warmup — 28
Where Our Eyes Go — 32
Color Your Chakra — 34
Mala — 44
Starting Anew Each Day — 52

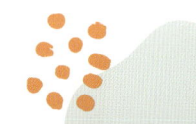

PART 2: CONTEMPLATION 55

Quieting the Mind	56	Knitter's Eight-Fold Path	70
Finding a Teacher	57	Opposite Thoughts	78
Listening to Your Body	58	Loving-Kindness	80
Knitter's Choice	59	Single-Pointed Focus	84
Finding and Exploring Our Edge	64	Resting Our Eyes	85
The Power of Silence	65	Making Space	88
Following Intuition	66		

PART 3: PRACTICE 91

Daily Repetition	92	Resets	102
Cravings	93	Work In Progress	104
Begin Where We Are	94	Knitting and Yoga Styles	105
One Stitch at a Time	95	Mental Flexibility	110
Sticking to It	96	Anytime, Anywhere	114
Impermanence	98	Transitions	118
Nonattachment	99	Finding Balance	120
Stash Status	100	Noticing One Thing	122
Giving Back	101	Taking Care	124

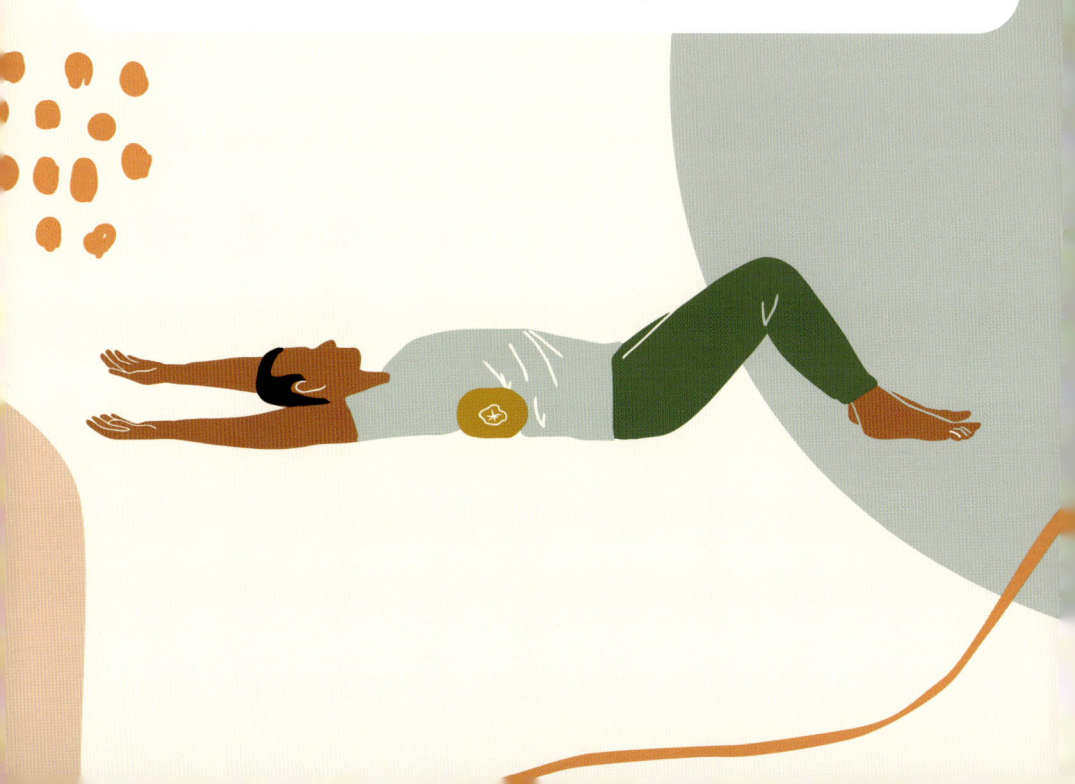

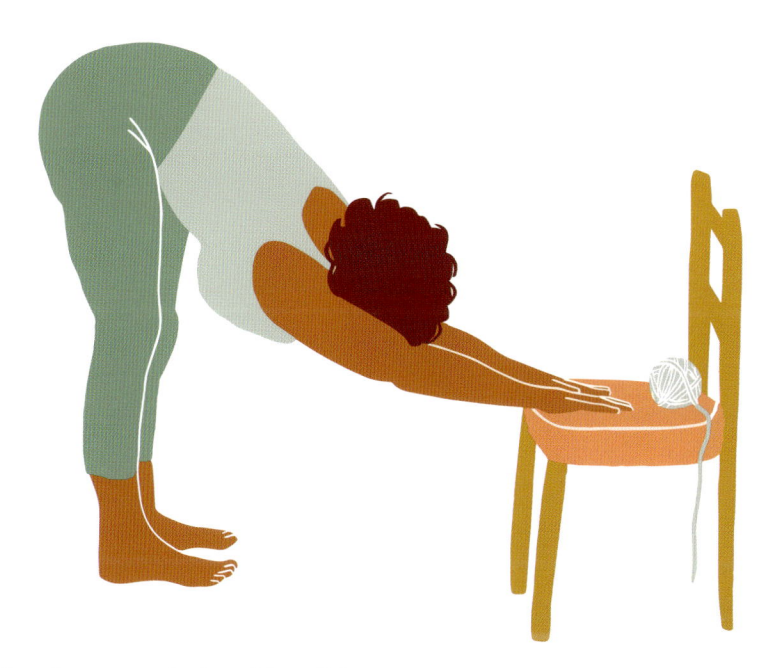

PART 4: JOYOUS ENDEAVORS 133

Life Force	134	Go Ahead and Laugh	154
Obstacles	142	Knitting with Tears	155
Inversions	143	Sun Salutations	156
Finishing	146	Knitflix	160
Contentment	152	Slow Mo	161
Control	153	Gratitude	167

APPENDIX 169

Index of Explorations	170	Further Reading	184
Basic Terminology	172	Acknowledgments	186
Basic Props	180	In Closing	186

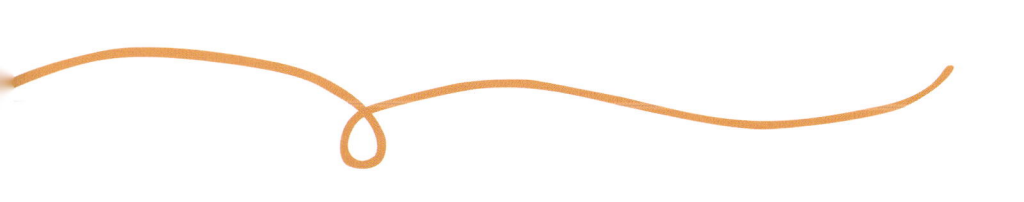

FOREWORD by Melanie Falick

A couple of years ago—during a period in my life that required a lot of public speaking—I realized that I had an effective remedy for the nervousness that inevitably struck me just before an event was about to start: The remedy was knitting, and it was literally at my fingertips.

When my heart began to pound and my thoughts muddled, I learned to pull out an easy project—or even just a swatch—and knit a few rows. Almost immediately I would feel my breathing rate slow and my heartbeat settle as my body and mind began to integrate. My anxiety didn't disappear altogether, but it lost its disruptive edge, and—with the help of just a few stitches—I was able to ground myself in the moment.

This was right around the time I started editing *Yoga of Yarn*, the book you are reading now, so I have to wonder if some of the wisdom of Liza Laird's manuscript was already seeping into my consciousness. Liza and I met via email—at the suggestion of our mutual friend, artist and author Heather Ross—then on the phone, then at my home. At that first in-person meeting, while we were talking about Downward Dog, my pup Sammy—as if on cue—extended his front legs forward and lowered his chest toward the floor, the exact movement that I have always assumed inspired this pose's name. It seemed like this relationship was meant to be.

During the two years that followed, Liza and I discussed and transmitted text and then layout files back and forth more times than I can remember, sculpting and refining this presentation to most clearly communicate the ideas Liza had begun to share with me (and Sammy) on that first day in my house. Liza understands that knitting, like yoga and meditation, can be a pathway to wellness, even more so when all three are combined. Her goal is to share the ways in which these symbiotic practices have helped her through her personal journey—from healthy youngster to yoga teacher to cancer survivor to mother to knitwear designer—and guide those of us who are interested in learning from her. She teaches us about beginning, setting intentions, finding ease and developing flexibility in both mind and body, channeling energy, tapping into intuition, and so much more.

What I may love most about this book is that you can open it to nearly any page and find a useful, accessible posture, perspective, or challenge. Or, if you prefer, you can read it page by page, front to back, from here to the end or vice versa. Liza's lessons make sense either way. She explains that we can begin our *Yoga of Yarn* journey anywhere, even with just a few moments of deep breathing, perhaps on a yoga mat or in a chair in a quiet area of our home or possibly while sitting in traffic or waiting at a doctor's office. Most important is repetition. Just like a handknitted sweater is made up of many stitches, each one formed using a distinct formula and part of a process we repeat over and over again, a yoga and meditation practice is made up of many intentional moments practiced consistently.

These days I meditate for five minutes every morning upon waking. At the dog park with Sammy, I do Reverse Prayer (page 27) and Eagle Arms (page 88) poses to open my chest and shoulders.

If I can't fall asleep at night, a few minutes of Alternate Nostril Breathing (page 139) or Ocean Breath (page 138) often helps. I like to flip around within this book and see what pops out at me.

I realize now that I can call upon my knitting to ground me not only as I prepare for a public speaking event, but also at other times when I feel off kilter or just need some space from the ups and downs of life. There have been periods in my past when I meditated for longer and when I attended multiple 90-minute yoga classes a week, and maybe I will return to that at some point. But for now I understand that I am where I am meant to be. The "perfect" practice is the one that I am engaged in right now, not the one I think I am supposed to be doing or the one my fit neighbor manages.

This is my practice. This is my yoga of yarn.

Melanie Falick is an independent writer, editor, and creative director. She is the author of several books, including *Making a Life: Working by Hand and Discovering the Life You Are Meant to Live.*

FOREWORD

INTRODUCTION

When I was young, I rarely had any aches or pains. I couldn't fathom that knitting might aggravate my body. After all, knitting was my go-to stress reducer. But at the age of 31, I found a golf ball–sized lump in my right breast. I had been trying to get pregnant for the first time, but instead of growing a life inside me, one of my cells had the gall to take it upon itself to grow uncontrollably without my consent. I was thrown into a slew of treatments to eradicate this cancer from my body.

In almost an instant, I went from being able to move easily and knit for hours to everything hurting all the time. Persistent inflammation, joint aches, and neuropathies—these are the side effects of my cancer treatment. Not to mention the general anxiety I felt about my surgery and chemotherapy. Suffice it to say my world, mentally and physically, entered a state of unrest.

For a decade before the cancer diagnosis, I had been studying and teaching yoga. I often found interesting ways to combine yoga with knitting, but back then I did not always appreciate the depth of the link between the two. When cancer upended my world, I tapped into yoga to try to manage my physical and mental anguish. I also explored how certain yoga poses and sequences could alleviate my pain and discomfort after long stretches of knitting. As time went on and my health improved, my focus broadened to yoga as a pathway to knitting with comfort, ease, and joy throughout all of life's ups and downs, as well as the natural aging process. This book is my best attempt to share my explorations with anyone who might benefit from them.

My passions for yoga and knitting started long before my battle with cancer. My mom taught me to knit when I was eight years old. I began meditating when I was eleven, and I started my yoga practice when I was fourteen. In college, the closest I ever came to rebellion was skipping class to knit a gift for a friend. After college, I moved to New York City to take a job in the marketing department of a large fragrance company. Before long I felt stifled there and would leave the office crying more often than you can probably imagine. As a young woman,

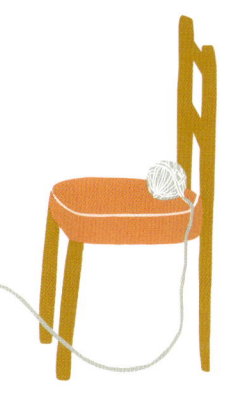

I felt an intense need to both prove myself and please people, both of which went into overdrive in the workplace.

To soothe my discomfort at work, I spent a lot of my spare time in formal yoga training. I earned teacher certifications from YogaWorks and Phoenix Rising Yoga Therapy. I trained as a life coach with the Coaches Training Institute. I began teaching locally. As I built up my class schedule and confidence in my ability to make a career out of what I loved, I took the leap and quit my day job. It scared me, but I did it anyway.

I increased the number of classes I taught at different studios around the city, and I rented a small space in Union Square where I offered private yoga and Phoenix Rising Yoga Therapy sessions. I also hosted yoga retreats out of town—as nearby as Vermont and as far away as Italy, Peru, and Thailand—and I guest-taught at studios around the United States. I loved traveling and teaching.

Eventually I launched Yoga + Yarn Retreats, multiday workshops for knitters interested in learning yoga, which I continue to offer to this day. The schedule generally includes a morning yoga class followed by a fun excursion. After lunch, we have another yoga session, then we work on our knitting projects together in the evening. One of my favorite parts of the Yoga + Yarn Retreats is our group dinners, where knitters from all over the world get an opportunity to forge relationships that last well after our long weekend together has ended.

After a few years of running my business solo, I met Kate Madden, a kindred spirit. At our first meetup, I joked that because we both loved yoga and knitting, we would obviously become best friends. Just as the words came out of my mouth, my dog, a feisty Shiba named Cosmo, memorialized the moment by peeing on her carpet. A fast friendship did, in fact, emerge, and after a few months, we decided to form Ragline Knits.

Together, under that umbrella, Kate and I now lead the annual Yoga + Yarn Retreats in Plymouth, Vermont, and Marfa, Texas. We also teach in-person and online workshops on a range of topics at the intersection of wellness

INTRODUCTION

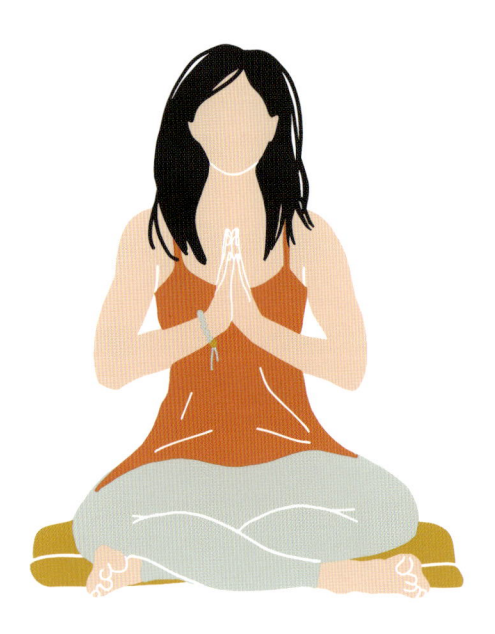

and crafting, among them Brioche as Meditation, Chair Yoga for Knitters, Knitter's Breath, and Bend, Stitch and Sip. Finally, we love designing new patterns. You can find our patterns in *Pom Pom Quarterly*, and on the Ravelry, Love Knitting, Craftsy, and Ragline Knits websites.

The yoga I write about isn't a fitness regimen. It's a lifestyle, one that I try to live and breathe all the time, with various degrees of success. It's a lifelong journey open to all of us—no matter who we are or what kind of physical shape we're in. Yoga embraces many concepts beyond the physical movements most closely associated with it, including meditation, as well as breathing exercises that help calm the mind and body.

It's a personal practice, and it's what you make of it. No one can tell you how to make yoga part of your life. The most anyone can do is make suggestions and share what works for them. In my personal practice, I like to let other people's suggestions wash over me and see how my mind and body respond to them. I try to listen to my own inner wisdom above all else.

My goal is to show you how easy it can be to incorporate yoga, meditation, and breathing techniques into your everyday life so that you are able to replenish yourself and come back to your center whenever your mind or body tells you something is off. Remember: When we care for ourselves physically, mentally, and emotionally, we become stronger and healthier and, consequently, better able to care for others.

I invite you to set *Yoga of Yarn* next to your knitting basket or drop it into your notions bag, then dip into it when you feel unease, when your body is asking you to listen to it, when your mind gets stuck in an unproductive pattern, or when it calls to you in any other way. Consider *Yoga of Yarn* your personal guide, a source you can rely on anytime, anywhere. As you try out these practices, listen to your body, explore your creativity, adapt as you see fit, and have some fun. Hopefully, the ideas I present here will invite greater ease and joy into your life for years to come.

Any errors you find in *Yoga of Yarn* are, of course, my own. Any benefits you extract from it are your own. They cannot exist without your willingness and participation. That's because this is not a book to read. This is a book to do and live.

With gratitude and love,

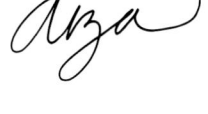

Liza

HOW TO USE THIS BOOK

You don't need any prior yoga experience to explore *Yoga of Yarn* and put it to work for you. All you need is a body, a chair, and a sincere willingness to care for yourself and try new things that will help you knit with greater ease.

I have divided *Yoga of Yarn* into four parts: Beginnings, Contemplation, Practice, and Joyous Endeavors. In Beginnings, I introduce some basic tenets of yoga and how they complement our knitting practice, including how to establish a beginner's mind, set an intention, and find ease. In Contemplation, I discuss concepts and techniques for quieting the mind. In Practice, I show how through non-attachment in conjunction with practice we can make yoga a way of life. Finally, in Joyous Endeavors, I explore different breathing techniques that can lead to perpetual growth, joy, and grace no matter what obstacles life throws our way.

Peppered throughout *Yoga of Yarn* are sutras—ancient threads of wisdom that form the foundation of yoga philosophy. *The Yoga Sutras of Patanjali* is the definitive guide to life as a yogi. Included here are the sutras I find particularly relevant for knitters. The sutras remind us that yoga does not just happen on a mat. It happens whenever we are open to the immense benefits it offers, including in the local yarn shop as we pick a new project, or while we make yarnover after yarnover.

Throughout *Yoga of Yarn*, I also invite you to try Explorations. Each Exploration is a step-by-step guide to a practice that builds flexibility of mind, body, and breath. You may wish to try each Exploration in the order in which I present it. Or you may prefer to skip around based on your body's needs on any given day. Regardless of how you explore, I suggest you arrive at each new concept with a Beginner's Mind (page 4) and Listening to Your Body (page 58).

There are six categories of Explorations: Yoga Postures, Mudras, Meditations, Breathing Practices, Yoga of Yarn Experiences, and Stitch Patterns and Practices. Each category has its own icon to make it easier for you to find. You can also find video demonstrations for Explorations at yogaofyarn.com.

As you put this book to work for yourself, you will no doubt find that what feels easy one day may feel hard the next, and vice versa. Meet yourself where you are in each moment without resistance, then let the practice do the rest of the work.

---

* *The Yoga Sutras of Patanjali* has been translated many times. My references are from the translation and commentary by Swami Satchidananda.

SiX CATEGORiES OF EXPLORATiONS

(See page 170 for an index of all 55 Explorations in *Yoga of Yarn*.)

Yoga Postures		Physical postures for you to explore on a chair, mat, or hard floor. Consult a doctor before practicing if you have any injuries.
Mudras		Hand movements to prevent or heal repetitive injuries and to introduce ways for the hands to channel energy.
Meditations		Mind-quieting mantras and meditations that explore yoga and knitting.
Breathing Practices		Breathing exercises that elicit a relaxation response, a sense of peace and calm.
Yoga of Yarn Experiences		Practices that explore the marriage of yoga and knitting to bring greater awareness to lived experience.
Stitch Patterns and Practices		Stitch sequences or techniques that bring attention to a specific connection between knitting and yoga.

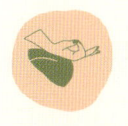

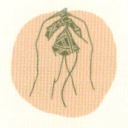

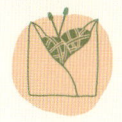

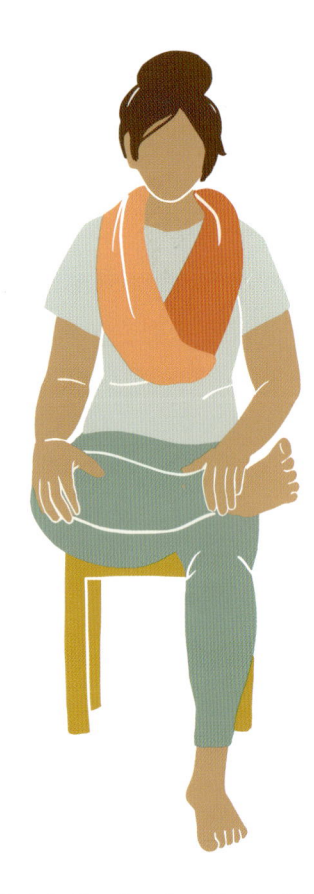

REST-AND-DIGEST

We exist in a world we do not understand and that can feel hostile to us. In each stage of our development, we encounter new fears, stresses, and anxieties—new risks to process, new threats to our continued survival and growth. The sympathetic nervous system enables us to respond when these situations arise by increasing our heart rate and sending blood to our muscles. It's the body's natural way of protecting itself in dangerous situations. This feature of the developmental program was extremely useful for early humans hoping to avoid becoming lunch for a pack of saber-toothed tigers. And it's still, of course, a necessary part of our survival mechanism.

But it is not without cost. It can become overactive. And our society often fosters this overactivity.

An overactive sympathetic nervous system leads to a host of other issues that plague our modern experience. Yoga and knitting help elicit a relaxation response that shuts down this system and activates our parasympathetic nervous system, taking us from fight-or-flight to rest-and-digest. The parasympathetic nervous system allows us to conserve energy, slow our heart rate, and take it easy. We don't have to go to a spa or a yoga retreat to activate the relaxation response. We can elicit it just by taking five minutes to engage in our favorite healthy calming practice.

So, ask yourself: How do I elicit a calm state for myself? Are the ways that just popped into my mind productive and sustainable, or do their returns diminish over time? Can I maintain their effectiveness in eliciting the relaxation response without creating other problems along the way? Some people may turn to food or alcohol to calm themselves down. These solutions often work well for a while, but then they can also create problems of their own.

I have found that yoga and knitting are healthy alternatives that keep on giving. I can embrace them for five minutes or five hours, and they do the job every time—they get me back to my center and ready to face the world as a contented, purposeful person.

This book is full of practices that engage the parasympathetic nervous system. Pick and choose the ones you like and let them become habits. One row of knitting. One minute of meditation as you wait for the bus. Alternate Nostril Breathing (page 139) or Legs Up the Wall Pose (page 144). These practices are nearly infallible as long as we call on them and incorporate them into our lifestyles. Even just a little bit each and every day goes a long way.

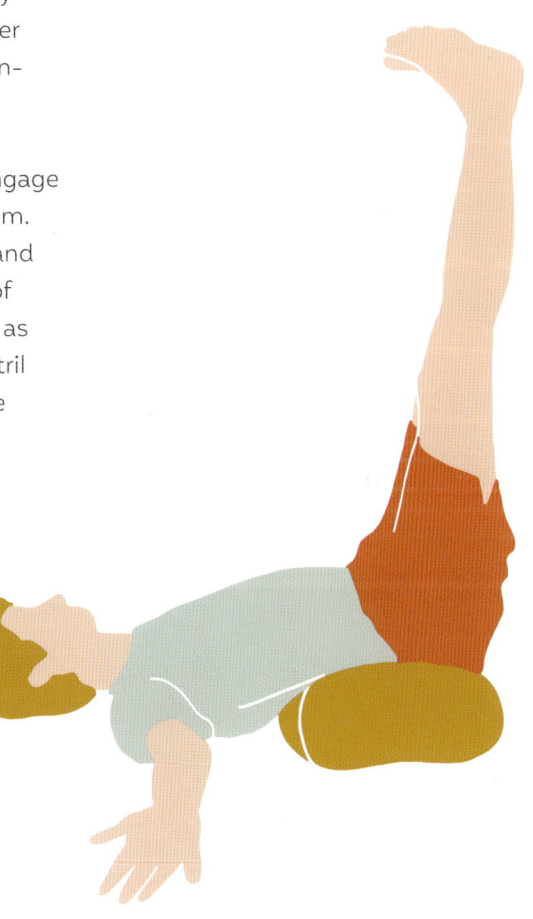

DEVELOPING A HOME PRACTICE

Incorporating yoga into our everyday lives means establishing a home practice. I have always favored my home practice over offerings outside my home because it gives me space to explore what intrigues and challenges me on my own terms. The same goes for my knitting. I can engage in a lot more trial and error and, in the process, figure out what I like and don't like. I can learn from my mistakes and successes at my own pace.

I am not discouraging practice in public settings. They offer unique benefits we often can't get when we're alone. Especially if we are just starting out on our yoga journey, being able to watch others take poses can be invaluable. Same with knitting. Getting tips from more experienced knitters in real time can accelerate our growth exponentially. And nothing beats a belly laugh shared among a group of knitters or connecting with a fellow knitter over a passion for a technique or project. Home practice is not a replacement for group practice, but it is a necessary component for growth.

If we aren't knitting or doing yoga regularly at home, we can start now. We can give it even just a few minutes each day. We can go slow as long as we are steady—daily repetition is key to our growth. Before we know it, we'll be plopping down in our preferred spot each day without even thinking about it. When we have a consistent home practice, it becomes easier to fit in our yoga and knitting anytime, anywhere. We are able to find our center wherever we may be.

ALL YOU NEED IS YOURSELF TO START A HOME PRACTICE, AND MAYBE A CHAIR. A LIST OF BASIC PROPS CAN BE FOUND ON PAGE 180.

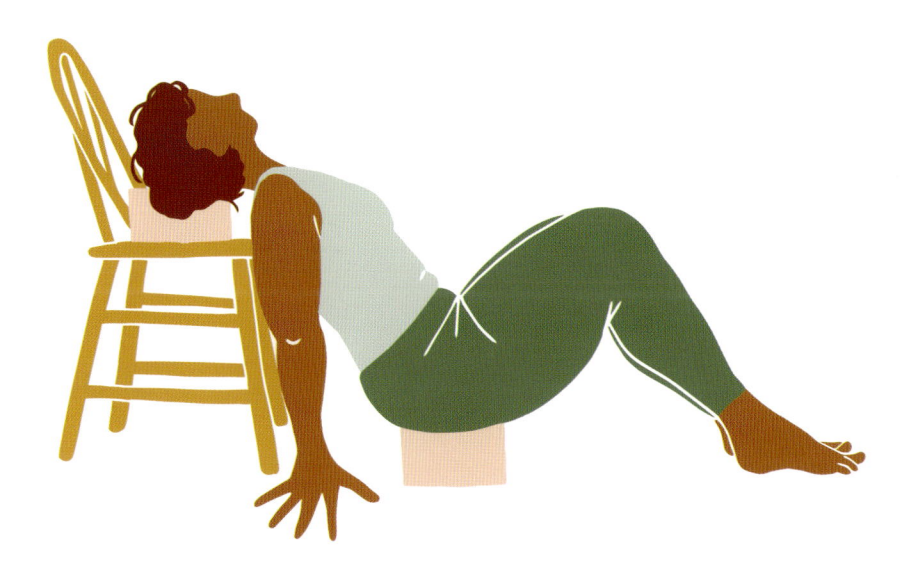

SACRED SPACE

Creating a sacred space within our home for yoga and knitting increases the odds that we will find the time to practice on any given day. We don't need to have our props out all the time, but it's nice to know we have a go-to spot to avoid putting yet another decision between us and our yoga or knitting. When I lived in NYC in a tiny apartment, I stored my yoga mat under the couch when I wasn't using it (and my yarn under my bed). Each and every day I placed my mat on the same spot on the floor and had the same routine to pull out my props and make time for my practice.

The goal is to put as few decisions as possible between ourselves and our yoga. If we must ask ourselves every day—*where am I going to practice?*—or, *where should I store my props?*—it becomes that much harder to establish a routine.

FIVE MINUTES TO START

A good way to get started is to set aside five minutes. Pick a meditation, a breathing technique, or two yoga poses to try out in a sequence. Turn on some music you like and set a timer for five minutes.

If you feel like stopping when the timer goes off, then stop. If you're feeling like five minutes wasn't enough, keep going. Especially in the beginning, never push yourself past your limit. When you begin to experience resistance, end the session. If you start resisting, just stop. You don't want resistance to prevent you from trying again tomorrow.

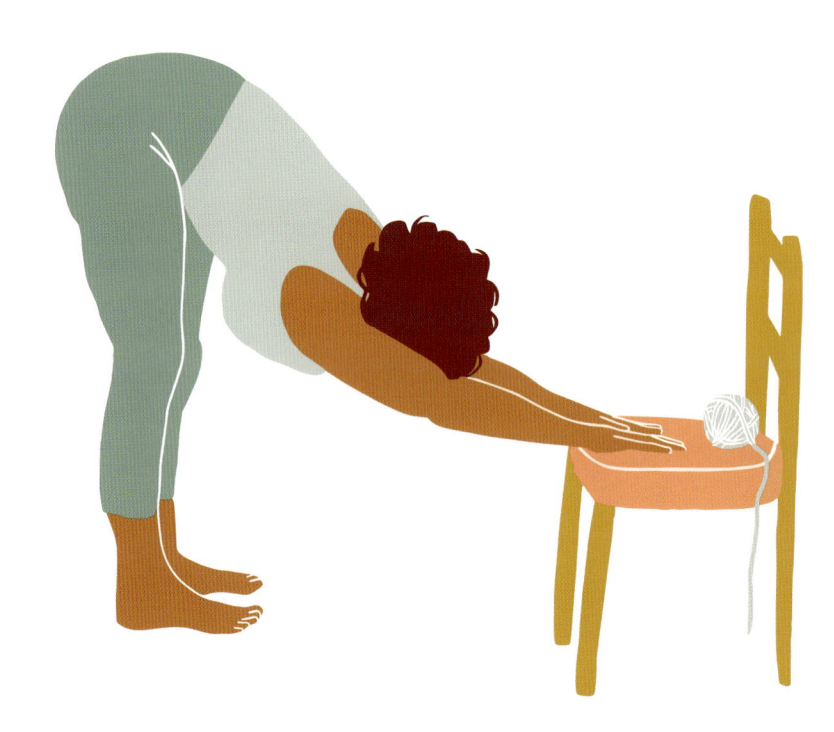

Remember there's no set length a yoga practice needs to last. Yoga classes at studios are generally 60 to 90 minutes, but five minutes at home, ideally in the same spot each day, can be just as beneficial. Remain realistic about your time commitment, and don't put pressure on yourself to do more. On some days your practice will naturally lengthen because the body will ask for it. After two to three weeks of reminding yourself to practice for five minutes each day, it will become a habit and the benefits will come. You will notice them if you pay attention. And they will probably make you want more.

If just reading about practicing every day feels overwhelming, start with every other day or once each week and slowly increase. Be easy on yourself and keep going!

> YOGA CLASSES AT STUDIOS ARE GENERALLY 60 TO 90 MINUTES, BUT FIVE MINUTES AT HOME, IDEALLY IN THE SAME SPOT EACH DAY, CAN BE JUST AS BENEFICIAL.

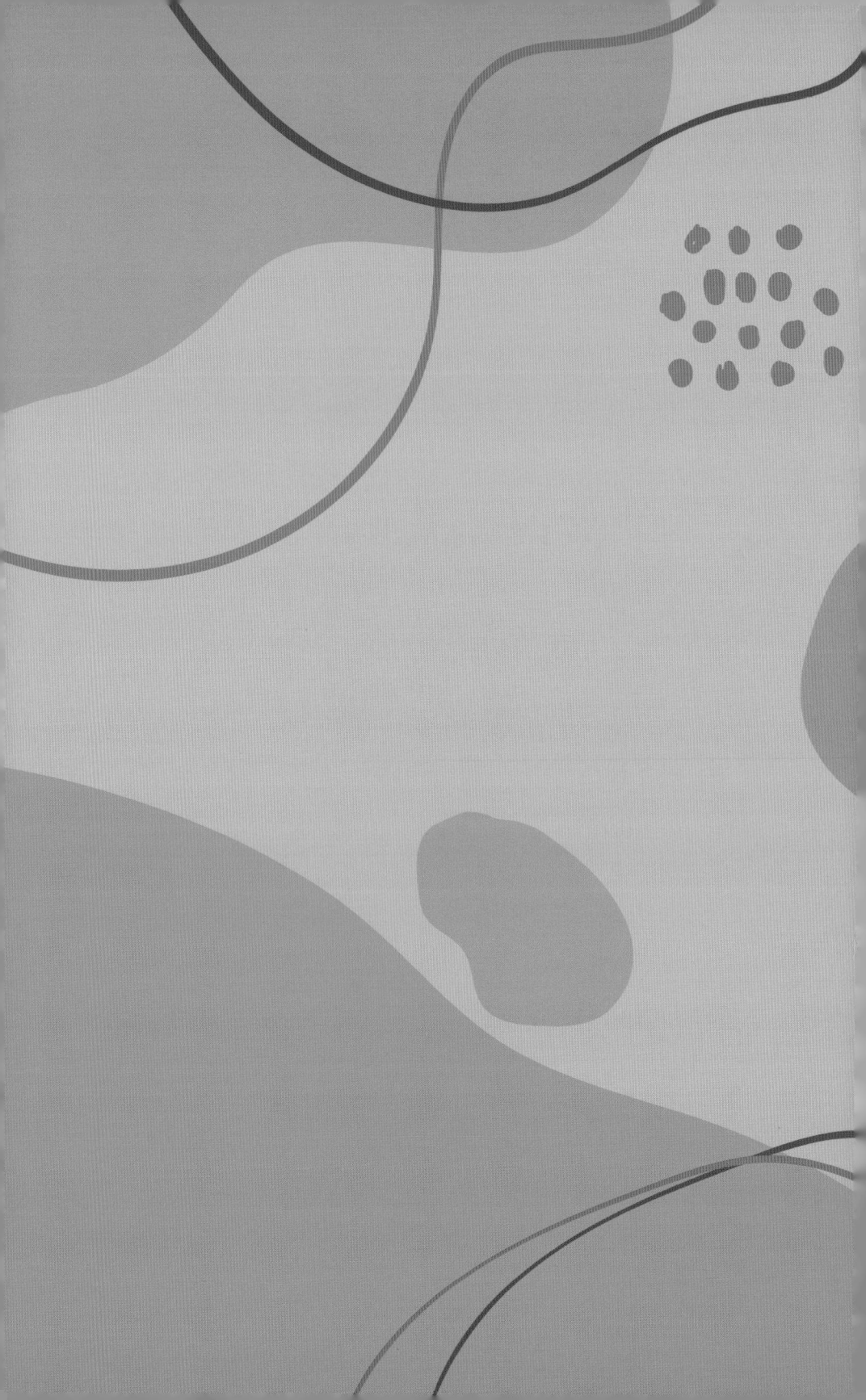

PART ONE

Beginnings

Let's begin with some basic tenets of yoga, including developing a beginner's mind, setting an intention, and finding ease, and explore how they complement our knitting practice. These are the cornerstones upon which a lifelong practice grows.

SUTRA 1.1

Atha yoganusasanam.
Now is yoga.

THE LIGHT WITHIN ME BOWS TO THE LIGHT WITHIN YOU.

NAMASTE

To begin, I say namaste to you. This Sanskrit word, pronounced *nah-mahs-tay*, loosely translates to *the light within me bows to the light within you*. Literally, *nama* means *to bow*, *a* means *I*, and *te* means *to you*.

In traditional Hindu culture, namaste is a greeting and sign of respect. In Western yoga, we have adopted this word to begin and end our yoga classes, often with our palms pressed together at the center of the chest and a gentle nod to those around us. The idea is that we are all honoring each other, our journeys, and our connectedness.

I honor the light within you and hope that as you explore *Yoga of Yarn*, you may find greater ease and light in your life.

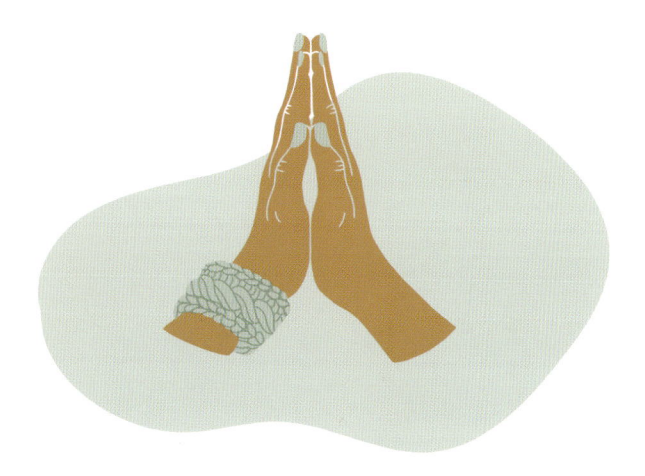

The first sutra tells us that right now is always the time to practice yoga—not a minute ago, not tomorrow. As long as we have open minds and remain willing, we can experience the benefits of yoga. So, let's dive in.

POWER OF THE UNIVERSE

Yoga and knitting have taught me that I can slow down, relax, and be present. And, most of all, they have taught me to believe in the power of the universe, to surrender to something far greater and more powerful than myself. The power of the universe is the all-knowing intelligence that governs you, me, and everything. Some call it God, source, spirit, or divine wisdom. It need not be a religious concept, but it most certainly is a spiritual one.

My experience has taught me that this greater power, which I choose to call the universe, has our best interests at heart, because we are part of it. That does not mean it's here to serve us. Quite the contrary. But it does mean we are its children and that we are part of its story.

INNER ENERGY

Begin by harnessing your own inner energy. It's real. It's physical. It's within us.

Benefits: Creates warmth. **Props:** None

1. Rapidly rub your palms together for about 1 minute.
2. Then, moving very slowly, pull the palms ever so slightly apart and feel the pulsing between them. That is your energetic body responding to a physical connection you've intentionally created.

If you don't feel it the first time, try a few more times, moving your hands apart more slowly.

A BEGINNER'S MIND REMINDS US TO BE OPEN AND TO RID OURSELVES OF EXPECTATIONS.

BEGINNER'S MIND

I was eight years old when I first learned to knit. I made a scarf. I was too young to have any preconceived notions about how it might go. I hadn't yet learned to fear looking silly or to compare my progress to others. I remember the joy of making something with my own hands and not worrying about what it looked like. That scarf had a lot of holes in it, and its shape was wonky, not exactly the rectangle it was meant to be. But it was mine, and I loved it. The act of making something without fear, preconception, or expectation was pure joy.

A beginner's mind reminds us to be open and to rid ourselves of expectations or comparisons. That seems to come naturally when we are young children, but as we age, we begin to evaluate ourselves in relation to others. While these protective skills can be useful at times, they also make it harder for us to learn new things. When I did my yoga teacher training, the instructor always reminded us to learn with a beginner's mind. Even if we had already learned the skill she was presenting that day, she asked us to pretend we hadn't and instead to learn it again anew—as a beginner.

When we approach our experiences with a beginner's mind, they become richer, more varied and complex, and worthier of our respect and appreciation. A beginner's mind assists us with our knitting and yoga in three ways.

1. FREES US OF JUDGMENT

When we learn a new stitch pattern or yoga posture with a beginner's mind, we are free of self-judgment. We stop worrying about how it *could* turn out. Instead, we provide space for our innate curiosity to take over. When a mistake becomes a curiosity as opposed to a failure, we can remain more present with each stitch or movement.

2. REDUCES ANXIETY

When I teach knitters or yogis a new skill, they often start off worried they won't catch on as quickly as they think they should. When we stop worrying about what we are able to accomplish on the first try, we save ourselves from unproductive anxiety.

3. SHUTS DOWN PROCRASTINATION

Many knitters lose some of their mojo when they face instructions that aren't immediately clear to them or at the end of a project when it's time to weave in ends. If we take a beginner's mind, we become more curious. We might study the stitches and discover something new about how they come together. We might reread the instructions to see if there is another way to interpret them.

I hope you approach this book with a beginner's mind. Don't assume you won't be able to meditate, open your shoulders, or make a super-stretchy cast-on. The beginner's mind lacks the power to acknowledge this kind of negative thinking.

Tell yourself now: *I will approach Yoga of Yarn with a beginner's mind.* You have taken the first step on your journey.

> WHEN WE LEARN A NEW STITCH PATTERN OR YOGA POSTURE WITH A BEGINNER'S MIND, WE ARE FREE OF SELF-JUDGMENT. WE STOP WORRYING ABOUT HOW IT COULD TURN OUT.

BEGINNINGS

SETTING AN INTENTION

Whether I'm starting a new yoga session or a new knitting project, I always set an intention to ground myself in the moment. Setting an intention allows us to manifest what we need in our lives at this very moment. Intentions are distinct from goals, which in general are about future plans. For example, my intention for this book is to share my experience of yoga and knitting with you, so you can incorporate their benefits into your daily life.

If you are setting an intention for a yoga class, you might say, *My intention is to bring ease into my life on and off the mat.* If you are starting to knit a blanket for a friend's baby, you could say, *My intention is to knit this project with love and compassion for the new little human who will be kept warm by it.*

While a knitting pattern tells you what stitches to make and where to do shaping, it doesn't tell you who to make it for or the purpose behind it. Yes, a vest is a piece of clothing, and a hat is an accessory, but there is more to a finished object than its classification. Perhaps you are making hats for chemotherapy patients, and you want to knit your compassion and prayers—or as I like to call them, good vibes—into the fabric. Or maybe you are making a cardigan for yourself, and your intention is to feel the pride you are knitting into it. Setting an intention at the beginning of the project makes explicit the part of your heart you want to bring to it.

> **SETTING AN INTENTION ALLOWS US TO MANIFEST WHAT WE NEED IN OUR LIVES AT THIS VERY MOMENT.**

An intention is tied to your personal feelings, values, and thoughts. It may come to you quickly, or it may not. If not, begin the process by asking yourself a few questions. Here are a few prompts to get you in the groove for a knitting project.

- Who am I making this project for?
- What do I want the recipient of the finished object to feel?
- How will knitting this nurture me?
- What do I appreciate about my knitting at this moment?

Based on these questions, here are some intentions that may resonate for you.

- I knit with ease.
- I knit love into each stitch.
- Knitting relaxes and soothes me.
- I knit peace, and I exhale tension.
- My knitting brings me joy.

Think of setting an intention as a tool to keep you grounded, at ease, and joyful. Or think of it like a yoga block that helps you hold a posture steady or go a little deeper. Once you get into the habit of setting intentions, you'll see that it is a handy tool available to you anywhere, anytime.

> AN INTENTION IS TIED TO YOUR PERSONAL FEELINGS, VALUES, AND THOUGHTS. IT MAY COME TO YOU QUICKLY, OR IT MAY NOT.

FINDING EASE

Finding ease doesn't mean making everything easy. It's about letting go and not resisting the flow of the forces around you. It's about allowing room for mistakes and having the humility to laugh about them. Sometimes when we are struggling or resisting, we aren't entirely—or even remotely—aware of it. We must be sensitive to our unease before we begin to find ease.

Bringing ease to a yoga posture is about letting go of resistance. You breathe into the pose and make gentle adjustments, so the yoga pose meets you where you are—as opposed to forcing you into discomfort. If your breath shortens or a body part trembles, back off a bit. Try Listening to Your Body (page 58) and allow yourself to rest when you need it.

Bringing ease to your knitting can come from softening the grip on your needles, releasing tension in your shoulders, or taking your time instead of rushing. Easeful knitting is the absence of resistance of any kind. Of course, knitting with total comfort and acceptance is easier said than done.

I recall a time when I got really excited about knitting a shawl with a combination of herringbone and brioche stitches, which together make a unique design with distinct textures. I started a swatch for it with a fingering-weight yarn and size 2 US (2.75 mm) needles, which were simply too small. For brioche, I always go down a needle size, and for herringbone, I always go up a needle size, which made it hard to get the size just right for this project.

Instead of accepting and laughing at this mistake, I chose to deny it and struggled to make the project work with the original needles. As the resistance built, I stopped paying attention to my posture and began forcing my yarn and needles together in an unnatural way. Eventually, I was resisting so much that I broke one of the needle tips right off.

> FINDING EASE DOESN'T MEAN MAKING EVERYTHING EASY. IT'S ABOUT LETTING GO AND NOT RESISTING THE FLOW OF THE FORCES AROUND YOU.

I put the yarn down and took a deep breath. I stepped away from the project and took a short break. When I came back to it, I reminded myself of my intention to knit with ease, saying the words out loud to myself a few times in a row.

I switched to larger needles and proceeded to knit a gorgeous swatch. Now every time I find myself resisting, I remind myself of what I call the Herringbone Incident.

EASE AS AN INTENTION

The beauty of setting an intention is that it has no inherent timeframe or expectation. It is a simple reminder of how you want to be in the world. The most important thing about setting an intention is to remain aware of it after you set it!

Benefits: Facilitates greater joy and less resistance. **Props:** Paper and pen

1. Take a moment to set an intention of ease for the day. For example, *My intention for the rest of this day is to bring more ease into my life and not resist the forces around me, whatever they may be.*
2. Write the intention down, and repeat it to yourself 3 times.
3. Keep this intention at the forefront of your mind throughout the day.
4. If you realize at some point that you have wandered from your intention, which is inevitable, take a deep breath and remind yourself by saying it out loud. Over time, it will become natural to recognize when you have been pulled away. Remembering to return to our intention fills us with a feeling of strength so long as we do not bring judgment to that experience.
5. When you are in bed at the end of the day, try to remember the sequence of events when you began to set your intention. Evaluate without judgment how well you kept the intention with you, and simply make a mental note.
6. When you wake up the next morning, set this or another intention again, and do the same thing in bed at night.

Do this for 5 days straight, then ask yourself how you feel. If this feels beneficial, it will naturally become part of your daily routine.

THE ART OF SITTING

We sit a lot these days—at a computer, in the car, on the subway or an airplane, waiting at a doctor's office, in our favorite knitting chair, on the couch watching television. No matter what we're doing, if we stay seated for long stretches, we create stiffness and tension in the body, particularly in the hips, neck, shoulders, and back.

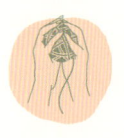

FIVE PRINCIPLES OF SITTING

Knowing how to position your body in the most supportive way will shape how you sit while knitting.

Benefits: Facilitates proper posture, relieves fatigue from sitting too long, and prevents injury. **Props:** Chair, folded blanket, blocks or books (optional)

Use extra support behind the back or under the hips if you have a back or hip injury.

1. Read through the Five Principles of Sitting and take mental notes as you go.

   Principle 1: Sit tall in your chair, maintaining the S curve of your spine. The S curve is the natural shape of your spinal column.

   Principle 2: Keep your knees at the same level as your hips, or lower. Use the blocks to help raise your hips away from the floor if necessary or, if you have longer legs, place a blanket underneath your hips to raise them.

   Principle 3: Lift out of your lower back. We want to avoid sinking into and rounding our lower back because that puts pressure on the spine and causes lower back pain and misalignment.

   Principle 4: Spread the collarbones and press the shoulder blades into the back to prevent slouching.

   Principle 5: Keep the chin parallel to the floor and slightly pulled back.

Paying attention to how we sit, as well as how long we sit, is the first step toward learning to sit in ways that keep the body and mind healthy. Slouching on the couch for long periods makes us feel sluggish and unmotivated. Sitting upright in meditation lifts our spirits. The more we think about how sitting affects our moods, the more attuned we become to the relationship between the body and the mind.

2. Take a moment to check in with how this positioning feels. Then take the blanket or towel and place it under your sit bones. Notice how it lifts your hips and protects your lower back. Sit like this for a few minutes. Consider whether this feels helpful or uncomfortable to you.

3. Place the blanket or towel behind your back to encourage your spine to straighten and your collarbones to spread. Sit like this for a few minutes. Does this feel helpful or uncomfortable to you?

4. Make a mental note of seated alignment that works for you. Next time you knit, set yourself up in this position before getting started. Refer to the Five Principles of Sitting each time you sit until the muscle memory builds.

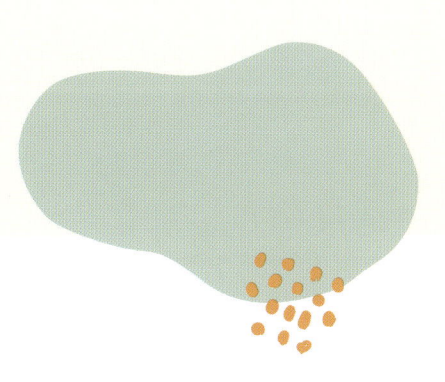

FLOOR SITTING

My favorite place to knit is sitting on the floor in Easy Pose with a cushion underneath me. I enjoy this pose because it allows my hips to open, my spine to lengthen, and my mind to find ease.

EASY POSE

Easy Pose, *sukhasana*, is a cross-legged position sitting on the floor. It is the most basic seated posture and a common position to start a yoga class or meditation. If you need extra support for the lower back, try sitting with your back against a wall.

Benefits: Activates rest-and-digest mode, relieves tension in hips, and improves posture. **Props:** Yoga block, folded blanket, or 1 to 2 pillows

If you have a hip, knee, or ankle injury, avoid this position.

1. Place 1 or 2 pillows, a folded blanket, or a yoga block underneath your bottom to lift your hips, so they are higher than your knees when you are sitting on the floor.
2. Cross your legs, right shin in front of left. Flex the feet to engage your lower leg muscles and protect the delicate knee joints.
3. Each foot will be underneath the opposite knee.
4. Straighten the spine, keep the chin parallel to the floor, and breathe evenly for 10 breaths. With a soft gaze, focus your eyes on a point on the floor about 3' (or 1 meter) in front of you.
5. Switch the crossing of the legs, and repeat with the left shin in front.

POSTURE CORRECTOR

Proper posture allows your spine to lengthen and your mind to be at rest. Sometimes a little nudge helps you reach that place of ease. A yoga strap encourages your chest to open as you practice.

Benefits: Eases the mind, spreads the collarbones, opens the chest, relaxes the shoulders, and improves posture. **Props:** 8' (244 cm) to 10' (305 cm) yoga strap

If you have a back or shoulder injury, skip this posture.

1. Sit in Easy Pose on the floor. Or, if you prefer, sit in a chair or remain standing. Make sure the strap is straight, not connected by the D-ring.
2. Place the strap behind you so it rests right below the tips of your shoulder blades, while holding the 2 ends in front of you.
3. Drape the ends of the strap over the shoulders and cross them behind you, so you can grab the opposite ends in either hand. You now have an X across the middle of your upper back and a strap end in each hand.
4. Pull on the strap ends. Either tie the straps in front of you under your breastbone or connect the D-ring and pull tight. You will feel your collarbones spreading and your posture straightening.
5. Try knitting a couple of rows in this position. Or simply hold the position for 10 or more breaths.

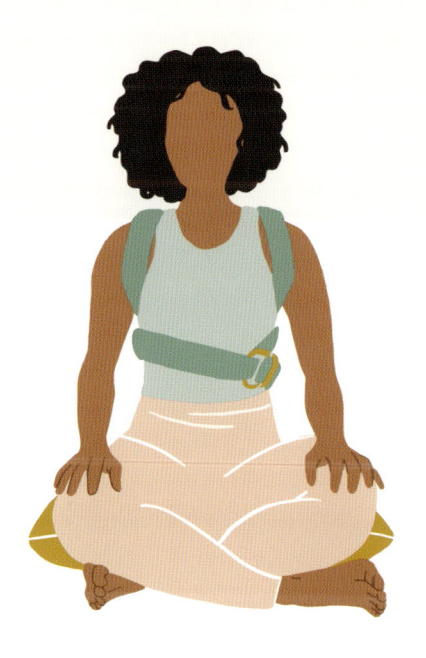

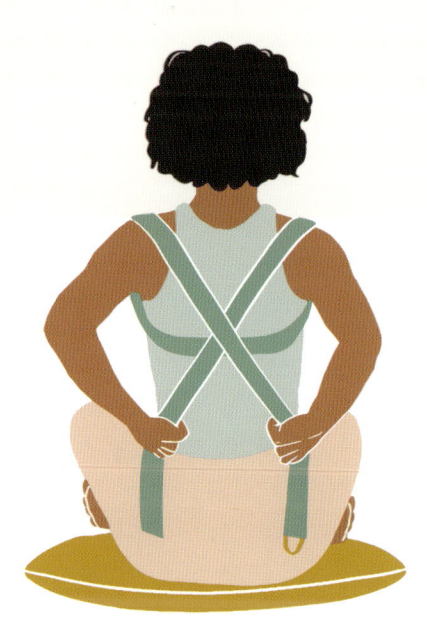

BEGINNINGS

STARTING WITH A STRONG FOUNDATION

Mountain Pose is the foundation from which all other standing poses evolve, in the same way that an appropriate cast-on represents a good start for all knitting projects. When we are in Mountain Pose, we are both strong and flexible, stable and steady. Some traditional styles of yoga will have you stand with your feet together. I recommend

MOUNTAIN POSE

Mountain Pose, *tadasana*, provides you with a chance to check in with yourself and evaluate the state of your body, mind, and breath.

Benefits: Improves balance, posture, and self-awareness. **Props:** None

Avoid this posture if you have a migraine or have difficulty standing for an extended period of time.

1. Come to a standing position, ideally barefoot. Place your feet hip distance apart. To gauge hip distance, lower your arms and reach both fists straight to the ground. The distance between your fists is hip distance. Wiggle your toes and look down at your feet. Adjust your feet so they are parallel.
2. Lift your gaze and keep your chin parallel to the ground.
3. Bend your knees a little and bounce ever so slightly. Sway your hips a bit. Roll out your shoulders, shake your arms.
4. Let your head turn side to side, open your mouth and stick out your tongue.
5. Roll your shoulders back and spread your collarbones.
6. Soften your front ribs in, so they are not sticking out. In other words, don't puff out your chest.
7. Release the tailbone toward the floor. Ground down into the earth with your heels and the balls of your feet. Lift and spread your toes, and then re-plant them into the floor.

feet hip distance apart, especially if you are not warmed up. It gives you more stability, and if your hips or hamstrings are tight, it gives you more space. Yoga is for all bodies, and it is important to pay attention to how your body reacts to poses so you can learn what works for you. Being aware is always the first step to learning yoga—and about ourselves.

8. Let all these movements subside, and stand tall with straight legs. Straight legs mean you are able to engage your upper thigh muscles and release them without difficulty. The muscles of the legs and buttocks are engaged yet not gripping.

9. Start to breathe in and out through your nostrils. Try deepening your inhales as you expand your abdomen.

10. Extend your exhales, releasing all that air out.

11. Continue standing for 3 to 5 minutes and notice the subtle movements of your body. You may see small shifts with each breath. Are you swaying from side to side? Do you find stillness and peace here?

Check out Retention of Breath (page 137), Ocean Breath (page 138), or Alternating Nostril Breathing (page 139) if you want to explore how to incorporate different breathing techniques into Mountain Pose.

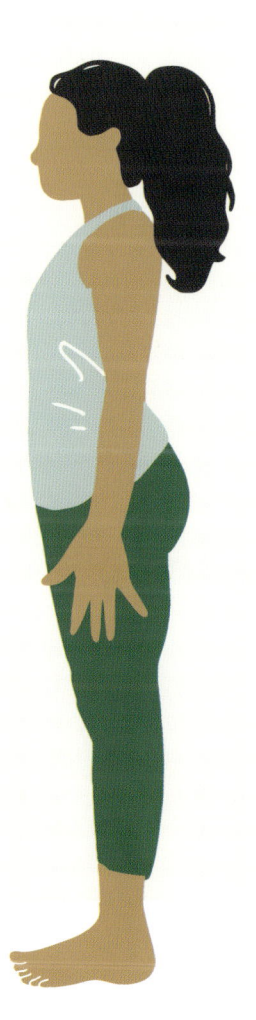

CASTING ON

As mentioned earlier, Mountain Pose is the foundation for all other yoga poses. If your foundation isn't strong, your ability to explore other postures will be compromised. The cast-on row is the foundation for all knitted fabric. If your cast-on isn't stable, your fabric may not do its job. For example, if you're working a hat from the brim up and you cast on too tightly, it may not fit around the head comfortably. If you are working a pair of socks from the cuff down and you cast on too loosely, the top of the socks may not hug the calf properly.

In my early years of knitting, I only cast on using the long-tail method. Now I know a bunch of different cast-on techniques and find that choosing the right one for each project makes all the difference. When I knit my first brioche cowl, I did a long-tail cast-on with a standard bind-off, and I found that the cast-on and bind-off didn't match as well as I would have liked. I still love that cowl as it was my first brioche project, but now I know that using the Tilly Buddy cast-on with Elizabeth Zimmermann's sewn bind-off would have been a better choice, because it mirrors the cast-on.

There are many different types of cast-ons, each with different pros and cons. If your pattern doesn't specify a cast-on—many don't—or you are knitting without a pattern, use your experience or the chart here to choose one. For your next project, consider trying a new cast-on to continue building a strong foundation for your knitting practice.

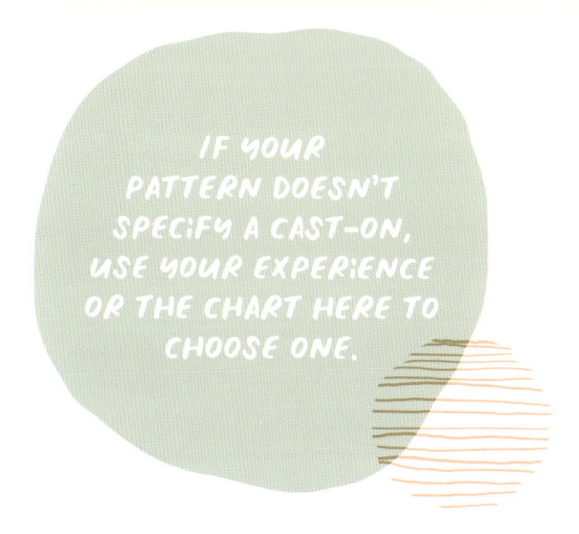

> *IF YOUR PATTERN DOESN'T SPECIFY A CAST-ON, USE YOUR EXPERIENCE OR THE CHART HERE TO CHOOSE ONE.*

YOGA OF YARN

Cast-On	Used For
Long-Tail	Almost any project. This is a versatile cast-on.
Tilly Buddy	Hats, socks, or anything that needs a stretchy beginning.
Backward Loop	In the middle of a row for an underarm or when you need something very elastic.
Tubular	Ribbing, hats, mittens, socks, and the wrist cuffs of sweaters.
Invisible Circular	Top-down hats, circular shawls, and blankets when you want a barely visible starting point.
Provisional	When you need live stitches to work later, such as for a border, or to do Kitchener stitch to connect two pieces of knitting without a seam.

FLOW

Many styles of yoga have predetermined sequences or patterns where postures are linked together in a particular order, but the term *flow yoga* is often reserved for a *Vinyasa yoga* class. In a *Vinyasa* class, we move from posture to posture deliberately and without a break in between. The sequence is designed with care and intention to foster a union of mind, body, and breath. Flow classes are fundamentally about breathing. We use our breath to support us through our movement.

As the body moves dynamically, the pace and timing of the breath aligns with the transition of the postures. If we find our movement and breath getting out of sync, we slow down the transitions to get our breath into alignment. We bring movement to our breath, not the other way around. As the breath and body align, we find our mind naturally integrates into the flow.

To me, knitting in the round, which doesn't require stopping and starting at the end of a row, is the knitting equivalent of *Vinyasa*. When I knit in the round, I get into a flow and easily reach a meditative state. My breath and hands align, while my mind focuses on the stitches. I find that I can achieve a similar state with back-and-forth knitting if the pattern has a concise and rhythmic flow.

> IN A VINYASA PRACTICE WE AIM TO ACHIEVE COMPLETE SYNCHRONIZATION OF MIND, BODY, AND BREATH.

KNITTER'S FLOW

No matter our age, it's important to keep our bodies flexible, or flowing, so we can move freely and without resistance. When our bodies are free of tension, our minds can be clear. Below is a short sequence of yoga movements linked with inhales and exhales to prepare the body to sit and knit.

Benefits: Increases blood flow and flexibility, sparks creativity. **Prop:** Chair

Avoid this practice if you have a shoulder injury.

Sit in a chair with feet flat on the ground. Take 1 breath per movement.

ARM RAISE
1. Inhale, raise your arms out to the side and up over your head.
2. Exhale, lower your arms to your sides.

SHOULDER ROLL
1. Inhale, roll the shoulders back.
2. Exhale, leaving shoulders in a neutral position.

NECK STRETCH
1. Inhale, tilt your head to the right, bringing your right ear to your right shoulder. Exhale.
2. Inhale, tilt your head to the left, bringing your left ear to your left shoulder. Exhale.

WRIST ROLL
1. Inhale, roll your wrists in 1 direction.
2. Exhale, roll your wrists in the opposition direction.

SEATED CAT-COW
1. With your hands placed on top of your upper thighs, inhale and arch your upper back slightly so the chest lifts toward the ceiling and your gaze lifts.
2. Exhale and round your spine like a cat, bringing your chin in toward your chest, shifting your gaze to your belly button.

Repeat the 5 poses a total of 3 times. Then begin knitting.

MEDITATION

Meditation is the engagement of contemplation or reflection. Through meditation we become more aware of and adept at managing our mental state. During meditation, we try to observe and quiet the mind by allowing thoughts to arise without latching onto them. Our thoughts become like passing clouds in the sky that move on before we can grab onto them.

For some, the idea of sitting still for a long time and focusing attention inward in this way seems difficult, scary, or just plain annoying. If that's you, forget about meditation for now, and simply trust that when you knit or do yoga, you are already on the path to meditation.

I was reluctant to meditate at first. I started to warm to the idea when I realized an obvious but underappreciated truth: Knitting is meditative by nature. The repetitive focus on stitches keeps the mind in the present moment. Similarly, taking a yoga class where another person guides us through a sequence of postures quiets the mind in a meditative manner. Listening to and trying to keep up with the instructor means we don't have time to get in our own way. Not getting in our own way is really the first step toward a robust meditation practice.

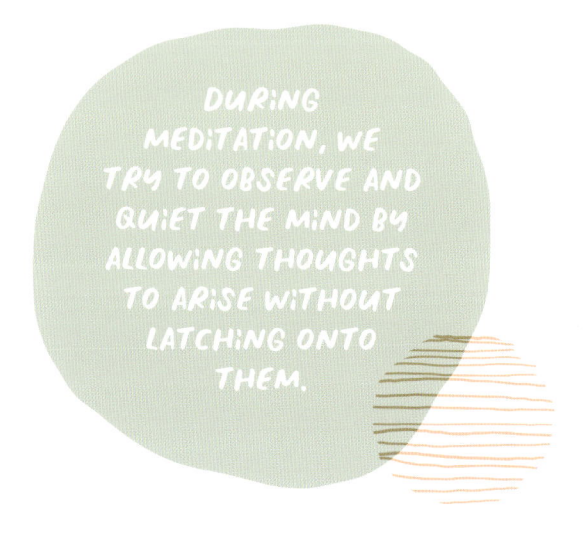

> DURING MEDITATION, WE TRY TO OBSERVE AND QUIET THE MIND BY ALLOWING THOUGHTS TO ARISE WITHOUT LATCHING ONTO THEM.

MANTRA

A mantra is any word or phrase repeated over and over. *Om*, the sound of the universe, is a widely recognized mantra. Many other Sanskrit words or phrases are commonly used as mantras, but English words work just as well.

Mantra meditation reduces stress and builds up mental clarity. And it's so easy! You simply sit or lie down and repeat a particular phrase.

> **MANTRA MEDITATION REDUCES STRESS AND BUILDS UP MENTAL CLARITY.**

You can build up your mantra practice anytime, anywhere—even while walking down the street or knitting. When knitting, I like to use my stitches as the mantra. When working a rib pattern, my mantra might be *knit, purl* across each row. If knitting lace, it might be *knit 1, slip 1, yarnover*, or whatever stitch pattern applies. Or, if my intention while knitting is to relax, I might repeat the word *ease* as I go. Choose mantras that work for you and your circumstances.

MANTRA MEDITATION

My first foray into meditation was through mantra. It was an easy way to start feeling comfortable in solitude. As you practice, notice when thoughts arise, and acknowledge their existence, but do not engage them. Each time your mind goes off track, bring it back to the mantra and let go. If you need to open and close your eyes a few times as a break, do so and then start again.

Benefits: Reduces stress and promotes clarity of mind. **Prop:** Timer

1. Seated or lying down, ground your body, set a timer for 1 minute, and close your eyes.
2. As you inhale, say *let*.
3. As you exhale, say *go*.
4. Continue this pattern for 1 minute.

Repeat each day, increasing the time, only as you feel comfortable doing so, until you reach 5 minutes per day without resistance.

MINDFULNESS

Mindfulness is the quality of being present in the moment without judgment. Mindfulness exists when we are fully immersed in what we're doing without attaching to it. Can you recall a time while knitting when you were entirely focused on the project at hand, tracking each stitch as it happened in that very moment? You were being mindful, likely without even knowing it!

> MINDFULNESS IS THE QUALITY OF BEING PRESENT IN THE MOMENT WITHOUT JUDGMENT.

Mindfulness meditation turns mindfulness into an explicit practice. It calls on us to focus on a particular point of awareness, like our breath. As thoughts, emotions, or sensations arise, we note them from a distance. We do not stray from our chosen focal point. We may start thinking of what to feed our kids for lunch. We don't fight that thought, but we watch it enter and move around our mind from a distance. We maintain that distance by keeping the spotlight of our attention pointed at our breath. Because we maintain distance, the kids' lunch has nothing to latch onto in the mind. That thought has no choice but to move on. (Hopefully, our kids eventually eat!)

Mindfulness meditation builds up a muscle memory so we can remain present no matter what life sends our way—good, bad, happy, sad, painful, or joyful. We watch these emotions come and go without attaching to them. The more we practice mindfulness meditation, the more we reduce stress and anxiety, cultivate clarity of mind, and facilitate love and kindness toward ourselves and others.

When you first begin exploring mindfulness, I suggest doing it alone at home when you know you will not be disturbed, if at all possible. I like to find space for mindfulness in the morning as I wait for coffee to brew. I start by exploring my sensory awareness and the sounds, smells, touches, and tastes that connect me to the world at this moment. I isolate the sound of the coffeemaker. I seek out the aroma of the coffee. I watch the drip as the coffee fills the pot. I notice the sounds and the colors. I imagine the taste. Throughout the day, I try to do the same thing when I'm doing the dishes, buying groceries, or folding my laundry.

There is no magic to mindfulness. You just try. You practice and observe your progress without judging it. You let time and repetition do the work for you. It all starts with a little willingness to try.

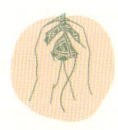

MINDFUL YARN

Read through all of the steps before beginning so you don't have to refer back as you try this practice. Then set a timer for 5 minutes.

Benefits: Reduces stress and improves clarity of mind. **Props:** Chair, ball of yarn, timer

1. Sit tall with a ball of yarn in your hands. Keep your eyes open for a moment and gaze at the yarn. Take a deep breath. Notice the color or colors of the strands. Feel the weight of the ball. Notice how thick or thin the strands feel.
2. Close your eyes and slide the yarn between your fingers. Notice the texture of the strands and the feel of the yarn on your skin. Gently place the yarn against the side of your cheek. Does it feel different?
3. Lift the yarn below your nose and inhale. What do you smell?
4. Let the yarn rest in your hands as you explore what you notice about the yarn.
5. Breathe gently for a few more moments. Then go about your day.

Repeat this practice each time you buy a new ball.

KNITTER'S MUDRAS

Mudras are symbolic ritual gestures. They form a seal between two body parts so energy can flow without restriction. Particular hand mudras are used in meditation and yoga to sharpen focus, activate creative flow, and tap into our inner wisdom. These mudras also strengthen the hands, preventing injury and relieving tension in tight spots.

> MUDRAS FORM A SEAL BETWEEN TWO BODY PARTS SO ENERGY CAN FLOW WITHOUT RESTRICTION.

When practicing a hand mudra, we hold our hands in a particular way to bridge our internal energy channels and move energy throughout the body. The way we hold our knitting needles is a mudra as well. When we hold our needles, they become an extension of our body. Our body's energy can

SALUTATION SEAL

The Salutation Seal, *anjali mudra*, is often referred to as prayer hands. The term *anjali* translates to offering, and this mudra is often paired with the phrase namaste.

Benefits: Stretches wrists and creates flexibility in chest. **Prop:** none

If you have a hand or wrist injury, avoid this mudra.

1. Seated or standing, press the palms of your hands together at the center of your chest. Press firmly so you feel your collarbones spreading.
2. Keep your palms pressing at the center of your chest for 10 breaths.
3. Experiment with lowering and raising your pressed palms. Inhale as you bring the base of your pressed palms up to your collarbones. Exhale as you bring your sealed hands down to where your fingertips are below your chest.
4. Shake out your hands.

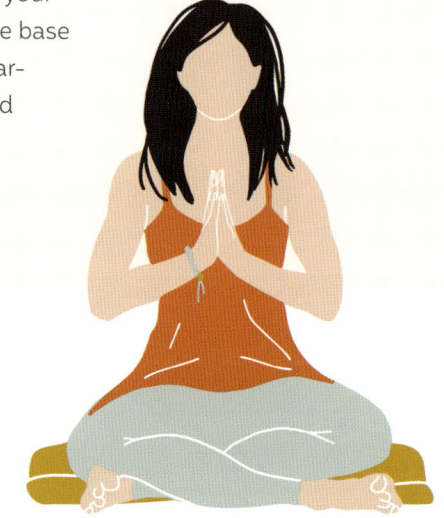

YOGA OF YARN

flow into them unrestricted in the same way that tennis players' racquets or golfers' clubs become extensions of their bodies.

Knitting daily can build up tension in the hands. the muscular equivalent of knitting the same stitch over and over again to create a bobble, a big ball of yarn that just sits in our body and wreaks havoc over time.

Find below four mudras I find particularly useful for keeping my hands healthy for knitting.

CONSCIOUSNESS SEAL

Try Consciousness Seal, *chin mudra*, as a short knitting break between rows. Do it for 10 breaths and then go back to knitting. Also use this mudra while meditating.

Benefits: Calms the mind, brightens mood, and boosts energy. **Prop:** Chair (optional)

If you have hand pain, avoid this mudra.

1. Sit comfortably on a chair or the floor.
2. Rest your hands on your thighs or knees.
3. Bring thumb and index finger together on each hand. Keep the other 3 fingers stretched out.
4. Face your palms toward the floor.
5. Take 5 to 10 breaths.

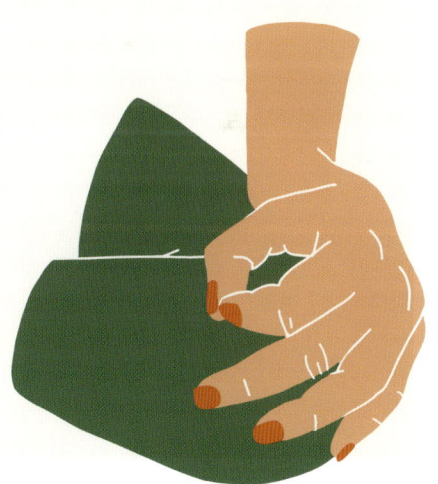

BEGINNINGS

CLASPED GESTURE

Clasped Gesture, *ganesha mudra*, opens the pectoral muscles and relieves stress. This mudra is named after *Ganesha*, a Hindu deity, known as the remover of obstacles, so it is often done when beginning something new. When doing this mudra, set an intention to remove any obstacles that might come up, before beginning a new knitting project.

Benefits: Opens the heart and relieves muscle tension around the chest.
Prop: Chair (optional)

If you have a hand or wrist injury, avoid this mudra.

1. Sit on the floor in Easy Pose (page 12) or in a chair.
2. Press your palms together in *anjali mudra* (page 24). Keeping your palms together, turn your hands so the back of your right hand faces your body and your fingertips move in opposite directions. The tips of your fingers face away from each other.
3. Start to slide your fingertips toward each other while curling your fingers and interlocking them together.
4. Hold this pose while taking a few deep breaths.
5. On an exhale, without unclasping your hands, gently pull your hands away from each other. You will feel an opening across your chest and arms.
6. Release the clasp and switch sides. Start in *anjali mudra* again, then turn your hands so the back of your left hand is facing your body, and your fingertips are facing opposite directions.
7. Pull your elbows away from each other as you begin to curl your fingers, hooking them into each other.
8. Take a few deep breaths, and on the exhales, without unclasping your hands, pull your hands away from each other.
9. Release and shake out your hands.

Repeat 2 times each side.

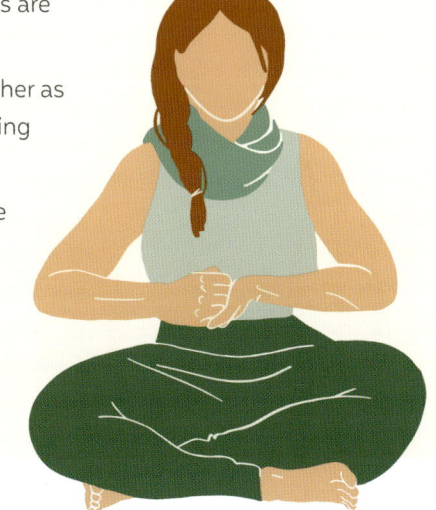

REVERSE PRAYER

Reverse Prayer, *paschima namaskarasana*, is an indispensable mudra for the avid knitter. It is similar to Salutation Seal (page 24), as both positions have the palms pressing together. However, this version has the palms pressing behind the back. If you can't press your palms together behind your back, have no fear! Start by holding opposite elbows or pressing your fists together. With frequent practice, eventually you may be able to press your palms together. Don't force it.

Benefits: Reduces tension throughout the body and mind. Opens the chest, shoulders, wrists, and forearms. **Prop:** Chair (optional)

Avoid this pose if you have a wrist, elbow, or shoulder injury.

1. Before attempting this posture, try a few neck and shoulder rolls to warm up the body.
2. While sitting or standing, stretch your arms out to the sides in a T shape.
3. Turn your thumbs toward the floor so your palms face behind you.
4. Bring your arms down behind your body and flip your fingers up toward your back to bring the palms of your hands together.
5. Allow the inhales and exhales to flow smoothly, without restriction. Take 10 deep breaths, and release flow in your hands down your back slowly shake it out.

Repeat a total of 3 times.

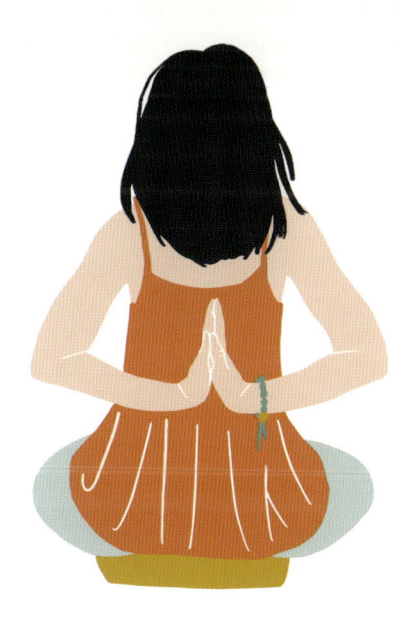

LiKE SWATCHiNG BEFORE WE KNiT A SWEATER, THiS WARMUP PROVIDES US WITH iNSiGHT THAT WiLL HELP US MOVE FORWARD PRODUCTiVELY.

WARMUP

Deep breaths and simple movements at the beginning of a yoga class awaken the body and mind, alert us to how we are feeling mentally and physically, and prepare us to transition into more advanced postures without strain.

During these initial movements, we may notice tightness or small aches and pains in the body. We may notice if our mind is centered or wandering. Sometimes we may feel wondrously serene, with Gumby-like flexibility. No matter where we fall on the spectrum, we take note of whatever we are working with that day.

A warmup is tailored to where we intend to peak. Many instructors tailor the warmup to the goals for the session. For example, if I'm leading a class with a split as the peak posture, then we'll start by warming up our hamstrings and hips. Our bodies tell us during the warmup if and when they are ready to try a half or full split. Some days that happens sooner, some days later, and some days not at all.

Although many knitters sit down to knit without a second's thought about their body's readiness, I highly recommend a regular warmup. Like swatching before we knit a sweater, a warmup provides us with insight that will help us move forward productively.

KNITTER'S WARMUP

These are easy stretches to eliminate unnecessary stress and prevent injuries to the shoulders, back, and wrists—the parts of the body we use most when knitting. Try them out on their own or all together. I like to do them before I start knitting and also during short breaks every 20 to 30 minutes. Keeping the body pain-free not only helps our knitting, it also helps us prepare to sit for meditation.

HAND SHAKE

Benefits: Relieves tension in hands and creates warmth. **Prop:** Chair (optional)

If you have a hand or wrist injury, avoid this practice.

1. With your arms by your side, bend your elbows so your hands come up toward shoulder height in front of you.
2. Shake your hands left to right, up or down, or both in an alternating pattern.
3. Shake for 10 seconds, then rest for 5 seconds.
4. Repeat a total of 3 times.

FIST TO JAZZ HANDS

Benefits: Strengthens the hands, lubricates finger joints, and increases range of motion to help you knit longer. **Prop:** Chair (optional)

If you have a hand, elbow, or wrist injury, avoid this practice.

1. Hold your arms out at your sides with your elbows bent against your sides.
2. Relax your shoulders and spread your collarbones.
3. Face your palms forward and your thumbs up toward the ceiling.
4. Make a fist and then release your hands so your palms are spread open and your fingers are stretching long.

Repeat 10 times. Gradually work up to 25 to 50 repetitions.

(continued on next page)

(continued from previous page)

ANKLE TO KNEE

Benefits: Opens the hips to relieve tightness from sitting for an extended period of time. **Prop:** Chair

If you have a hip or knee injury, avoid this practice.

1. While seated in a chair, scoot yourself forward so your bottom rests at the edge of the seat.
2. Plant your feet firmly on the ground.
3. Lift your left leg and open the hip out to the left. Raise your left ankle and place it on your right thigh, just above your right knee. Keep your left foot flexed to protect your left knee.
4. Stay upright or, for a deeper stretch, lean forward over your legs as your spine lengthens. Place your left hand on your inner left thigh and your right hand on your right quadriceps (upper thigh). Come forward as far as you can without feeling any pinching or pain in your knee or hip. Be sure to keep your spine straight so you don't hunch.
5. Take 5 deep breaths.
6. Move slowly out of the posture, then switch sides and repeat.

Repeat a total of 2 times per side.

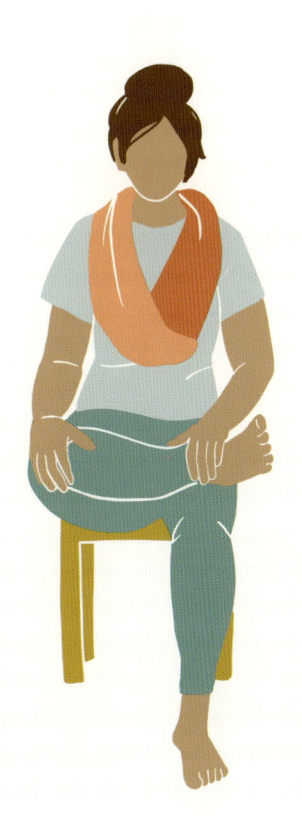

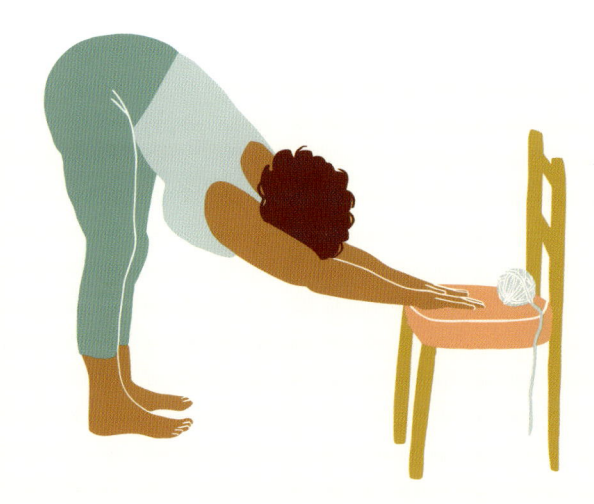

SUPPORTED DOWNWARD FACING DOG POSE, *adho mukha vrksasana*

Benefits: Releases tension in the shoulders and neck, lengthens the back of the body along the spine and backs of the legs, and opens up the shoulders and back. **Props:** Chair, table, or wall

If you are unable to invert or have a shoulder, back, or hamstring injury, avoid this practice. If your shoulders' range of motion is limited, use the wall and start with the hands above the head, walking your feet back and lowering your hands to create more space only when you feel comfortable.

1. Stand facing the front of your chair. Place your hands on the top rail of the chair. If the chair is not very stable and you feel like you might push it over, place your hands on the arms or seat. Or, if you have a table nearby, put your palms flat on top of it, shoulder distance apart.
2. Walk your feet back until they are directly underneath your hips. Root your hips into the chair.
3. Move your shoulders away from your ears. Relax your head. Feel your hips stretch away from the chair or table, lengthening your spine.
4. Take a few deep breaths here. Bend one knee at a time. Shift your hips from side to side. This will open up the sides of your body as well.
5. Stay in the pose for 10 to 20 breaths.

Repeat a total of 2 times.

> SETTLING INTO OUR DRISHTI IS THE FINISHING TOUCH TO DISCOVERING A WELL-BALANCED MEDITATIVE STATE IN ANY POSE.

WHERE OUR EYES GO

When knitting, we keep our eyes on our stitches, especially for intricate patterns. In yoga class, when holding a posture, we choose a specific spot where our eyes can focus to enhance concentration and balance. Yogis refer to this focus, or gaze, as *drishti*. We try to keep our *drishti* soft so that our eyes relax, which we know is happening when areas near our focal point enter our peripheral vision. Settling into our *drishti* is the finishing touch to discovering a well-balanced meditative state in any pose.

Of course, it's easy to let the eyes wander during yoga class—to look around at what other people are doing or wearing or watch what's happening outside. When that happens, we have to remind ourselves to stop searching. The more we practice, the more quickly we notice when we're drifting and the more quickly we can refocus our eyes on our *drishti*, knowing the mind will follow. With lots of practice, we may also learn to notice that we are about to drift away before we actually do. We may even build up such strong concentration muscles that we are able to maintain our *drishti* as long as we choose.

KNITTER'S GAZE

If you incorporate this simple exercise into your knitting routine, you will soon find that you are meditating each day whether you intend to or not. It makes taking the next step to establishing an explicit meditation practice that much easier.

Benefits: Improves concentration; fosters a pleasant rhythmic connection between your mind and the yarn flowing through your fingers. **Props:** Current knitting project

1. As you knit, notice where your gaze is pointing. Do your eyes wander every few stitches?
2. Set an intention: *I will point my drishti to my stitches as I create them.*
3. Knit with this gaze and intention for 10 minutes. Observe what happens without expectation or judgment while reminding yourself every so often to maintain soft eyes.

> THE MORE WE PRACTICE, THE MORE QUICKLY WE NOTICE WHEN WE'RE DRIFTING AND THE MORE QUICKLY WE CAN REFOCUS OUR EYES.

COLOR YOUR CHAKRA

Chakra is the Sanskrit word for wheel or disk. These wheels are the main energy centers in our bodies and correlate to our levels of consciousness. Each one is associated with a different color. The wheels start at the base of our spine, corresponding to our most primitive level of consciousness, and go straight up the spine to the highest level of consciousness at the crown of the head.

By looking at our chakras, we can develop a deeper understanding of ourselves. When one chakra is out of balance, we may need to adjust something in our lives to get it back in alignment.

Each chakra is associated with a color and a set of qualities. The first wheel is the root chakra, *muladhara*, represented by the color red. The root chakra is related to our survival and safety needs. When this chakra is balanced, we feel grounded and stable.

The second wheel is the sacral chakra, *svadhisthana*, and is associated with the color orange. The element of this chakra is water, and it evokes a sense of fluidity. When *svadhisthana* is balanced, you have grace, acceptance, and compassion toward yourself and others. It allows us to go with the flow.

Moving up the body, we find the third chakra, the solar plexus, *manipura*, whose color is yellow. This wheel is the core of our physical, mental, and energetic bodies. This internal strength is what gives us the self-confidence to live to our fullest potential.

The fourth chakra is the heart chakra, *anahata*, associated with the color green. Opening this disk connects our body and mind, teaches us to love ourselves, and deepens our relationships with others. Bringing our awareness to opening the heart and deepening the breath allows for

> **CHAKRAS ARE THE MAIN ENERGY CENTERS IN OUR BODIES AND CORRELATE TO OUR LEVELS OF CONSCIOUSNESS.**

Chakra	Color	Location	Qualities	Knitting Project	Yoga Pose
Root, *muladhara*	Red	Base of spine	Security, safety	Yoga socks	Tree (page 38)
Sacral, *svadhisthana*	Orange	Below navel	Creativity, sexuality	Skirt	Goddess (page 39)
Solar plexus, *manipura*	Yellow	Solar plexus	Confidence, wisdom	Belly wrap	Reverse Tabletop (page 40)
Heart, *anahata*	Green	Heart	Love, compassion	Sweater	Camel (page 41)
Throat, *vishuddha*	Blue	Throat	Communication, truth	Cowl	Fish (page 42)
Third Eye, *ajna*	Indigo	Middle of the forehead (third-eye point)	Intuition, foresight	Eye pillow	Child's Pose (page 42)
Crown, *sahasrara*	Violet	Top of the head	Understanding, spirituality	Meditation cushion	Seated meditation (page 43)

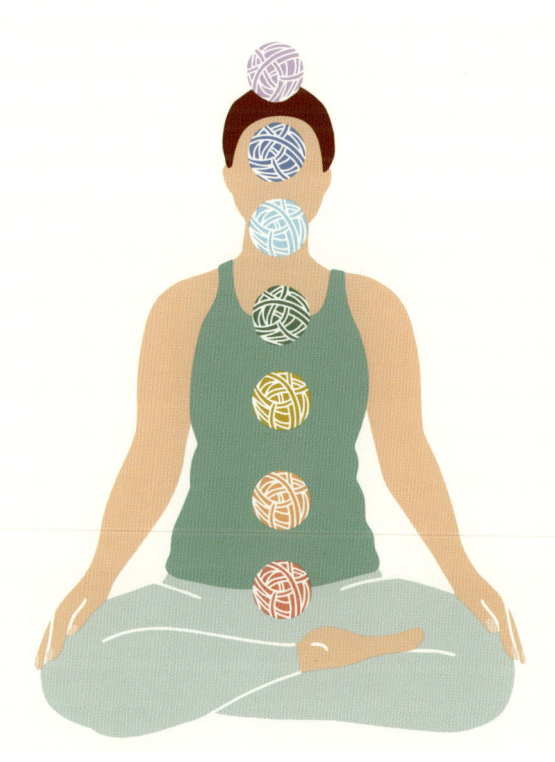

BEGINNINGS

> THE INTENTION YOU SET AND THE COMPASSION YOU SHOW YOURSELF AS YOU KNIT WILL HELP YOU WORK THROUGH WHATEVER IS OUT OF BALANCE.

expansion and union within. The energy and strength of the heart stems from its power to integrate and balance the mind and body through the breath.

We then move up the body to the throat chakra, *vishuddha*, where the color changes to blue. This chakra is about communication and our ability to express ourselves. When this wheel is balanced, we share our truth with ease and appreciate that there is no wrong way to communicate. Perhaps we communicate through song, dance, art, or knitting. We all have our own unique way to reveal our true selves.

The sixth chakra is the third eye chakra, *ajna*, and its color is indigo. This energy center is linked to our intuition and ability to see. We see not only through our eyes, but also through our own ability to trust our intuition.

Violet is the color of the seventh chakra, the crown, *sahasrara*. This chakra rises above the purely physical levels of understanding that ground the other wheels. It's located at the crown of the head and, when balanced, represents the cosmic consciousness—our ability to experience unity and understand that everything is connected at the most fundamental level.

Each of these chakras can be in or out of balance at any given time. To bring a chakra into balance, we can meditate with our *drishti* (page 32) on its location, color, or meaning. We can also look to our knitting. If you're not feeling grounded, making a pair of cozy red yoga socks might harmonize your root chakra. If your communication needs a little boost, you could knit a blue scarf to protect your voice and remind yourself to use it. The intention you set and the compassion you show yourself as you knit will help you work through whatever is out of balance.

A version of *Color Your Chakra* was originally published in the August 2020 issue of *Knotions Magazine*.

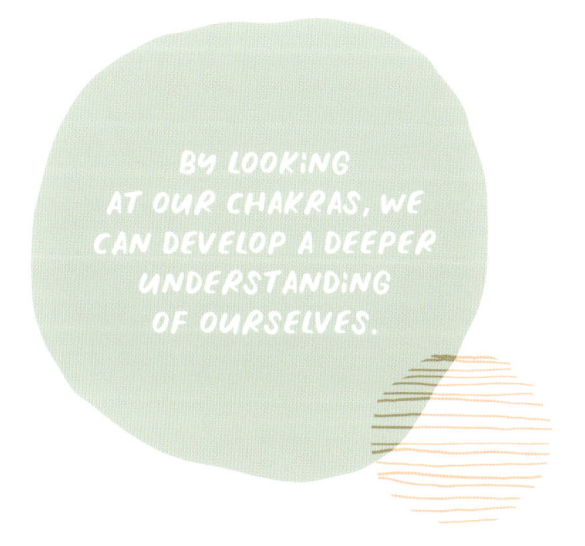

> BY LOOKING AT OUR CHAKRAS, WE CAN DEVELOP A DEEPER UNDERSTANDING OF OURSELVES.

CHAKRA BALANCING IN A CHAIR

This sequence builds upon the concepts and practices we have already explored. It's designed to create space in the body parts that get tight from knitting while exploring your chakras in a restorative manner. Try each of the 7 poses consecutively for a 30-minute chair yoga practice. Or try each individual pose at a time to take a 5-minute break from knitting.

TREE POSE, *vrikshasana*

Benefits: Opens the hips, body, heart, and mind, improves balance, creates stability, and activates rest-and-digest mode. **Props:** Chair, timer

If you have hip, knee, or ankle pain, avoid this posture.

1. Stand next to the chair with your left hand resting on the back of the chair for support.
2. Turn the right leg out from the hip and place the ball of your foot on the ground. Lift up your heel and rest it on your leg above the ankle. This is a kickstand position.
3. If you are struggling with strength or balance, stay here in kickstand for about 2 minutes then go to step 5.
4. Glide the sole of your foot up the leg so it presses against the side of the calf muscle. Stay here or try moving the foot higher until it is above the knee and pressed up against the inner thigh. Avoid placing the foot near the knee. Hold your foot at its highest comfortable point for 2 minutes.
5. Repeat on the other side and hold for 2 minutes.

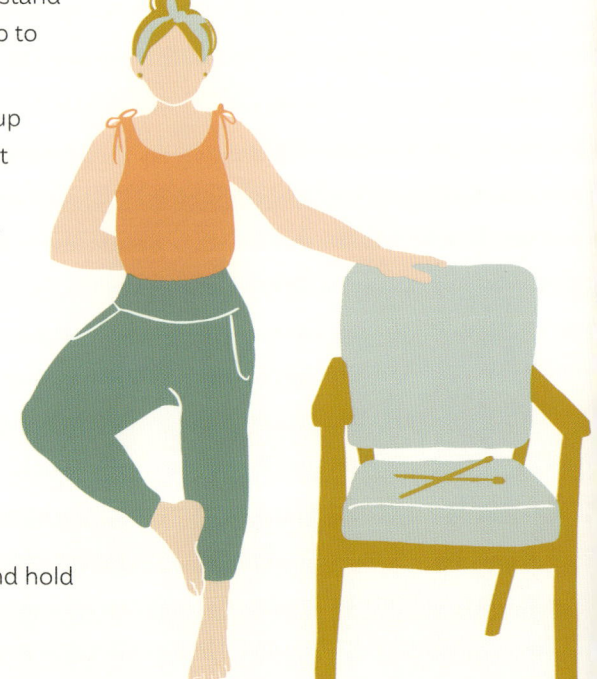

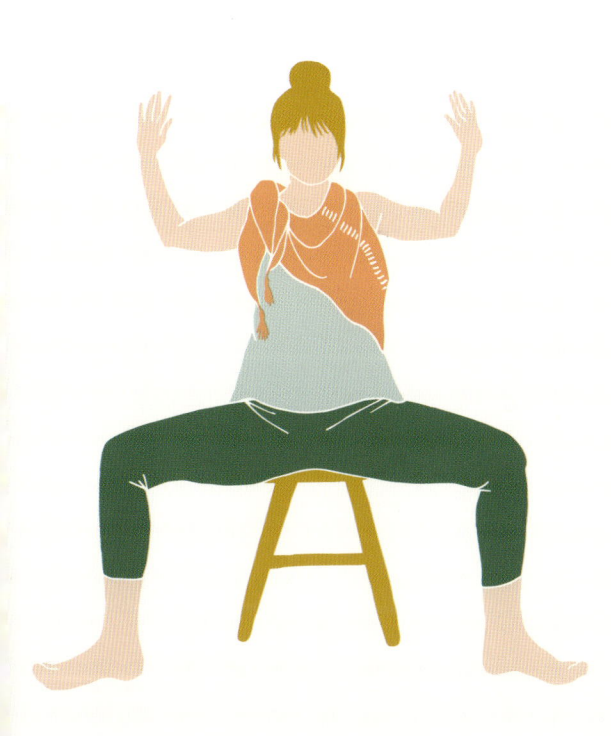

GODDESS POSE, *utkata konasana*

Benefits: Cultivates creativity and opens the hips and chest. **Props:** Chair, timer

If you have hip, knee, or ankle pain, avoid this posture. If you have shoulder or rotator cuff pain, leave your arms by your sides.

1. Sit on the center of the seat.
2. Spread your legs open as wide as you can. The legs should be bent with knees over ankles and feet turned out slightly so your toes point away from each other.
3. Take a deep inhale as you reach your arms overhead. Feel the entire spine lengthen.
4. Slowly move the elbows down and out to the side, stopping at shoulder height.
5. Turn the palms of your hands up toward the ceiling and tilt the pinky finger sides up as the thumb sides turn toward the floor.
6. Breathe steadily here for 5 minutes.

(continued on next page)

(continued from previous page)

REVERSE TABLETOP, *ardha purvottanasana*

Benefits: Strengthens the abdomen and the muscles along the spine, opens the hips and chest, and inspires confidence. **Props:** Chair, timer

If you have wrist pain, avoid this posture.

1. Sit on the edge of the seat and place your hands behind you, gripping the front of the seat.
2. Ground your feet, checking that your ankles are directly under your knees.
3. Press your hands down and lift your hips, lengthening your buttocks toward your knees.
4. Breathe in this lifted position for 2 minutes and then gently lower down.

Repeat a total of 2 times.

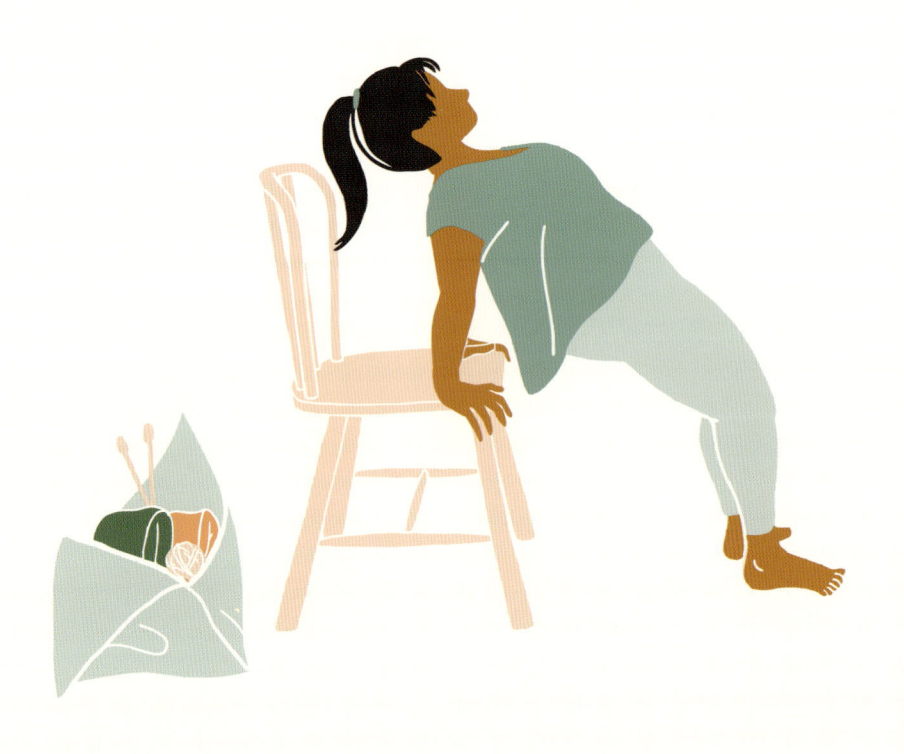

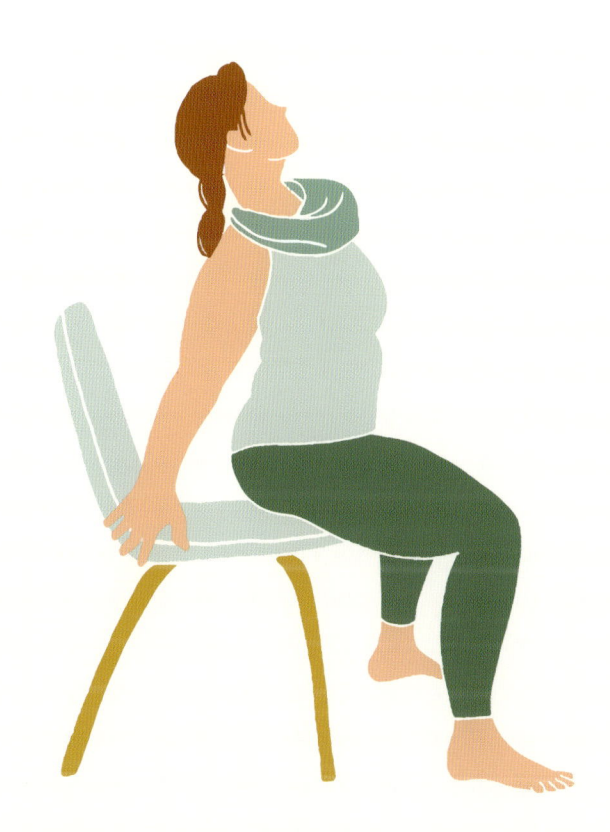

CAMEL POSE, *ustrasana*

Benefits: Improves posture and spinal flexibility while reversing the effects of rounding the back while knitting. **Props:** Chair, timer

If you have back pain, avoid this posture.

1. Sit on the edge of the seat with your feet hip distance apart.
2. Bring your hands behind you and grab the sides of the back of the chair.
3. Spread your collar bones and bring the shoulder blades together, creating a bend in the upper back.
4. Keep your chin parallel to the floor for a few breaths, then gently tilt the chin toward the ceiling as you lift your gaze up.
5. Breathe steadily here for 2 minutes.

(continued on next page)

BEGINNINGS

(continued from previous page)

FISH POSE, *matsyasana*

Benefits: Opens the muscles of the chest, relaxes the neck, and creates flexibility in the spine. **Props:** Chair, yoga block, 2 blankets or towels (optional), timer

If you have neck or back pain, avoid this posture.

1. Place a block on its lowest setting in front of the chair. The height of the block may need to be adjusted depending on the height of your chair. Place a blanket on the seat of the chair if desired.
2. Sit on the block with your back to the chair, knees bent, and feet flat on the floor hip distance apart.
3. Place your hands by your sides and lean back until your upper back and head are resting on the block and blanket behind you.
4. Drape another blanket over you, if desired. A blanket will help to warm the body so your muscles relax.
5. Bring your arms over your head and bend your elbows so your arms are resting on the chair behind you. The arms can also rest by your sides.
6. Breathe steadily here for 5 minutes. Come out of the posture as slowly as possible by scooting gently to one side and pressing yourself up to standing.

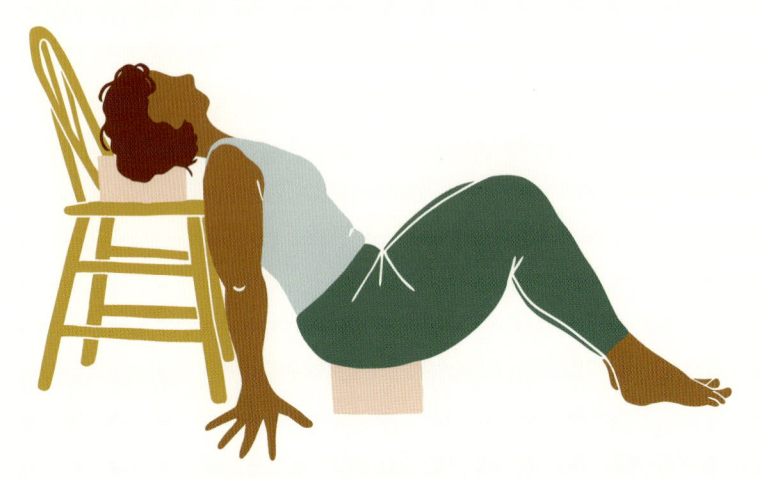

CHILD'S POSE, *balasana*

Benefits: Lengthens the back, opens the hips, and relaxes the mind. **Props:** Chair, 2 folded blankets or towels (optional), timer

If you have back or knee pain, avoid this posture.

1. Sit on your knees, facing the front of the seat of the chair about half an arm's distance away. Check that your knees are hip distance apart and your big toes are touching behind you.
2. Place a folded blanket between your calves and hamstrings.
3. Lean forward, stack your forearms on top of one another, and place your forehead on your arms.
4. Rest here for 5 minutes, switching the stacking of your forearms halfway through. If desired, place a folded blanket on the seat of the chair for comfort.

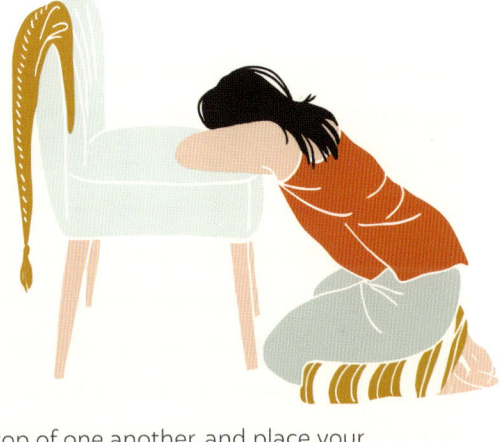

SEATED MEDITATION, *dhyana*

Benefits: Relieves gripping in the hips, improves concentration, and sparks creativity. **Props:** Chair, 2 folded blankets or towels, timer

If you have hip pain or if sitting for extended periods of time causes discomfort, do this lying down on your back.

1. Place a folded blanket on the seat of the chair and drape another one over the back of the chair.
2. Sit on the blanket on the chair and rest your tall spine against the folded blanket on the back of the chair.
3. Either place feet hips distance apart on the floor or cross your legs in Easy Pose on the chair.
4. Close your eyes or set a soft gaze on the floor about 3' or 1 meter in front of you. Allow the breath to find a steady, unforced rhythm. Relax your jaw.
5. Become aware of the sounds around you. Bring attention to your third eye. Place the middle finger of your left hand gently on the point at the center of your forehead. As your mind wanders, bring the awareness back to third eye. Notice the sensations that pop up as you sit in stillness. Release the hand to your lap, and where you need a reminder to focus the attention at the center of your forehead, place your fingertip back on the third eye. Meditate here for 5 minutes.

BEGINNINGS

MALA

Over the years, I have gathered many notions to support my craft—from multiple sets of interchangeable needles to various styles of cable needles and stitch markers. When I first started meditation, I also gathered some props that helped me transform it into a daily practice, including mala beads.

A mala is a necklace-like cord strung with 108 beads, usually made of seeds, nuts, crystal, or gemstones. Some people wear malas around their neck; others believe a mala must be hidden in a pouch. For many, a mala serves as a reminder of one's love or devotion to a particular person or idea. There are also mala bracelets, typically with 27 beads. There's no right or wrong with malas.

When used in meditation, malas are guides that help us to maintain focus and remember where we are in our sequence, just like a stitch marker does in knitting. There are a number of theories as to why 108 is considered an auspicious number. I like this one: 1 stands for the universe, 0 stands for humility in our spiritual practice, and 8 stands for infinity and timelessness.

No matter what meaning you do or don't ascribe to the number, it serves as a tool for you to frame your meditation practice. If you ever wonder how long you should meditate, you can use the 108 beads as a reference point. I usually try to complete at least one full circuit of 108 beads in each session, but it's really yogi's choice. You can divide the 108 beads into four sections of 27 beads each and make that your session length to start.

Picking your mala beads is like selecting your knitting needles. There are so many different kinds of stones, nuts, seeds, and colors to choose from. Touch and feel different kinds, and notice which ones move you. My first mala was made of turquoise, and I just love its look and feel. When I was traveling in India, I picked up a mala made of *rudraksha*,

> FOR MANY, A MALA SERVES AS A REMINDER OF ONE'S LOVE OR DEVOTION TO A PARTICULAR PERSON OR IDEA.

seeds that ward off negative energies. I find their bumpy texture stimulating between my fingers as I meditate.

To use mala beads for meditation, place them in your left hand. Locate the guru bead, the largest bead connecting all the other beads. Hold the guru bead between your thumb and third or fourth finger. Now move the beads one by one along your fingers in sync with either your breath or repetition of your mantra.

There are countless variations on this practice. For instance, some people prefer to hold the mala in their dominant hand. Some like to hold the other hand to their heart while expressing a loving intention for the meditation. No matter what variations you explore, always come back to the rhythm of repeating your mantra or regulating your breath as you move each bead between your fingers.

> PICKING YOUR MALA BEADS IS LIKE SELECTING YOUR KNITTING NEEDLES. THERE ARE MANY DIFFERENT KINDS OF STONES, NUTS, SEEDS, AND COLORS TO CHOOSE FROM.

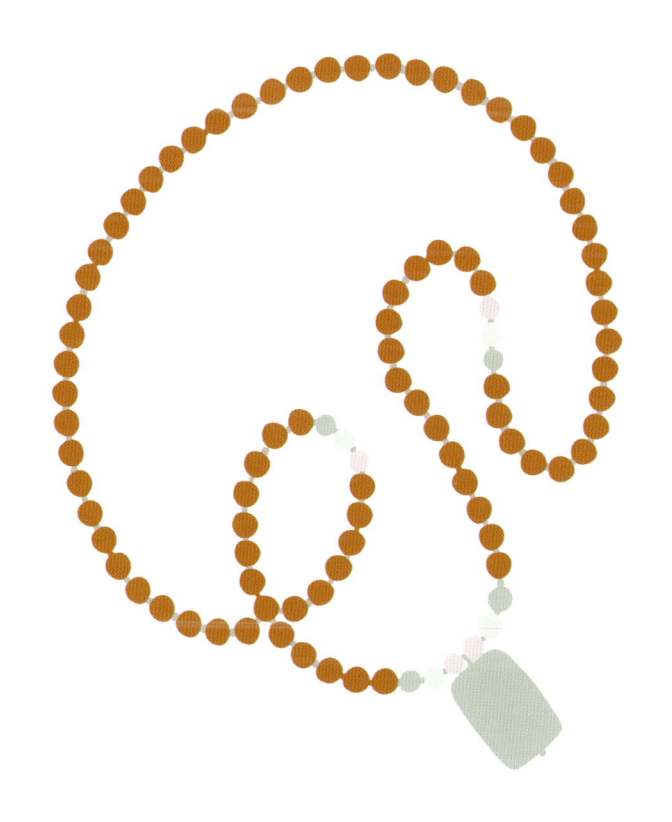

BEGINNINGS 45

BRIOCHE MALA COWL

One reason I love brioche stitch in the round is because it is rhythmic and requires a meditative focus. It reminds me so much of meditation with a mala. In this Exploration, I invite you to knit a brioche cowl using my Mala Cowl pattern. Consider combining this Exploration with the next one, Mala Cowl Meditation. Together they meld many of the concepts and practices we have been developing in Part 1.

When I first tried to teach myself how to do the brioche stitch, I struggled. The flow of the stitches eluded me. To embed it in my mind and body, I found I needed to knit 2 to 4 rows of brioche each day. As I repeated the stitches verbally and physically, the pattern eventually started to make more sense. By sneaking in even 5 minutes of knitting here and there almost every day, brioche became a part of my muscle memory, and now I find it more soothing than even garter stitch. The beauty of knitting and yoga for me is that I don't need to spend hours each day. The tiniest bit done on a *daily* basis yields enormous benefits over time.

I created the Mala Cowl pattern with 108 stitches to represent the 108 beads of a mala. With this cowl, the analogy I made earlier between beads and stitches is made literal. The stitches *are* our beads as we knit in the round.

Meditation is nonlinear. We aren't going from start to end in a straight line. We are going around in a flow that connects beginning and end and, in so doing, forces each to be melded into the other. Eventually we lose awareness of where we started and where we are going, and we become more focused on the precise moment of the journey as we travel it.

The cowl will wrap two times around the neck or hang like a long necklace.

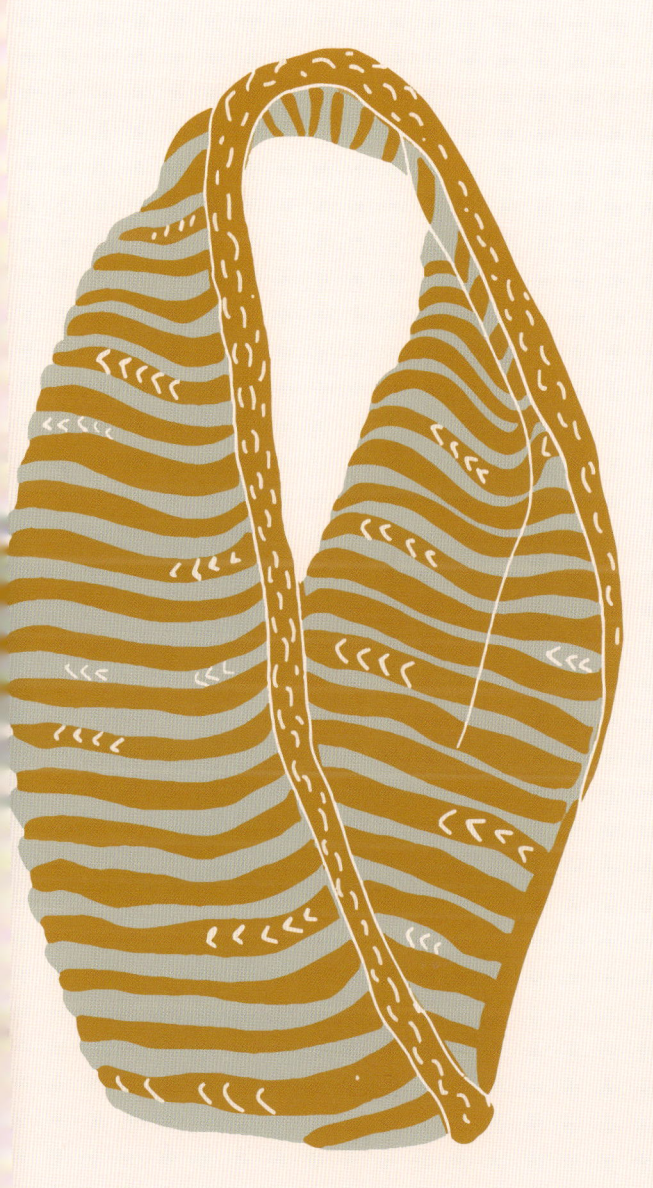

Size & Dimensions

13.5" (34.5 cm) wide (laid flat) by 8" (20 cm) tall (flat, unstretched)

Materials

2 colors DK weight yarn, 100 yards (92 meters) each

Size US 6 (4 mm) 16" (40 cm) or 24" (60 cm) circular needle, or size needed to obtain gauge; size US 8 (5 mm) 16" (40 cm) or 24" (60 cm) circular needle

Stitch marker

Gauge

16 stitches and 28 worked rounds (14 visible rounds) = 4" (10 cm) in Brioche stitch, using smaller needle, after blocking.

Always use a needle size that will result in the correct gauge after blocking.

(continued on next page)

BEGINNINGS

(continued from previous page)

Cowl

Using larger needle and yarn B, cast on 108 stitches with Long-Tail Cast-On. Join in the round, being careful not to twist stitches. Place a marker at the beginning of the round.

Knit 2 rounds.

Switch to the smaller needle.

Set-Up Round: With yarn A, *knit 1, sl1yo; repeat from * to end, bringing yarn back under the needle to the front after working the last sl1yo.

Round 1: With yarn B, *sl1yo, brp1; repeat from * to end.

Round 2: With yarn A, *brk1, sl1yo; repeat from * to end, bringing yarn back under the needle to the front after working the last sl1yo.

Repeat Rounds 1 and 2 until piece measures 7.75" (19.5 cm) from cast-on edge, ending with Round 2. Cut yarn A.

Switch to the larger needle.

Next Round: With yarn B, *knit 1, brk1; repeat from * to end.

Knit 2 rounds.

Bind off all stitches using Elizabeth Zimmermann's Sewn Bind-Off or your preferred stretchy bind-off.

Weave in the ends and block.

Glossary

Brk1 Brioche knit 1: Knit the stitch that was slipped in the previous row together with its yarnover.

Brp1 Brioche purl 1: Purl the stitch that was slipped in the previous row together with its yarnover.

Sl1yo Slip 1, yarnover: Before a knit 1 or brk1, bring yarn under needle to the front, slip 1 stitch purlwise, then bring yarn over needle to the back before working the next stitch (this will create a yarnover when the next stitch is worked); when worked before a purl 1 or brp1, slip 1 stitch with yarn in front, bring yarn over needle to the back, then under needle and to the front again to create a yarnover before working the next stitch.

TIPS FOR BRIOCHE STITCH

1. It takes knitting a few rounds of brioche before you can see the pattern. Have patience. It will look funky for a bit.
2. A brioche knit stitch (brk1) is when you knit a stitch and its yarnover together.
3. A brioche purl stitch (brp1) is when you purl a stitch and its yarnover together.
4. When counting stitches, the knit (or purl) stitch and its yarnover are counted as a single stitch.
5. Because of the slipped stitches in brioche, each stitch in a column of stitches will represent 2 worked rounds; keep this in mind when checking round gauge in brioche.
6. When you put your knitting away for a bit, be sure to work a few stitches of the next round so that when you come back to pick it up, you can read your stitches to see if you are on a brk or brp round.
7. At the end of each round, make sure both yarns are at the front of the work.
8. At the end of Round 1, make sure you work a yarnover on top of the last slipped stitch, ending with the yarn in the front of the work instead of in the back.

Elizabeth Zimmermann's Sewn Bind-Off

This sewn bind-off gives you a stretchy edge and mirrors the cast-on edge of a Long-Tail Cast-On.

1. Cut yarn tail to about 4 times the circumference of the edge you are binding off. Thread the tail onto a tapestry needle.
2. Thread the yarn through the first 2 stitches on the lefthand needle purlwise, leaving stitches on needle.
3. Thread the yarn through the first stitch again knitwise and slip the stitch off the needle.
4. Repeat Steps 2 and 3 until you have 1 stitch remaining on your lefthand needle. Thread the yarn purlwise through the last stitch and slip it off the needle.

MALA COWL MEDITATION

You can explore this moving meditation (page 174) whenever you sit and knit. Always remind yourself of your intention, and start your deep breathing with your feet on the ground before you pick up your needles. As you knit and repeat your mantra, you may find that your attention starts to wander. You may begin to think about dirty dishes or laundry. There's no need to stop your knitting and tackle those tasks, so remind yourself that you are here now to knit as a moving meditation. Let the thoughts flow and bring yourself back to your stitches.

Benefits: Increases concentration, calms the mind, relaxes the nervous system, and creates a foundation for your home knitting meditation practice.

Props: Knitting pattern, needles, yarn, notions, eyeglasses, water or tea, pen and paper to take notes for your pattern and write down your intention

1. Select a location where you know you can sit with a tall spine, focus, and relax without interruptions.
2. Place your supplies within easy reach. Turn off your phone or at least set it to *Do Not Disturb*. If helpful, put your phone in a different room.
3. Review your pattern to confirm that you understand the instructions and have all the supplies. I like to highlight areas where I know I'll need to pay close attention, such as when switching needles.
4. Choose the length of time for your meditation session by picking the number of rounds you'll knit. There's no required amount of time. Perhaps you'll decide that knitting a single round of 108 stitches is enough meditation for the day.
5. To begin the meditation, place your feet flat on the floor, straighten your spine, and spread your collarbones wide. Take a few deep breaths in through your nose and out through your mouth, exhaling as fully as possible.
6. After a few deep breaths, let your inhales and exhales steady, then start to breathe in and out through the nose. Then ask yourself what your intention is for this project (page 6). Setting an intention is about creating a mood—what you want to feel while you knit.
7. Write down your intention or repeat it to yourself a few times. Take deep breaths that fill your abdomen as you inhale, and empty your abdomen completely as you exhale. Allow your inhales and exhales to ground and prepare you for this new endeavor.

8. While casting on, continue to breathe consciously, staying aware of your inhales and exhales as you knit.

9. Once you have cast on 108 stitches, start to get into the flow of the pattern. Using each stitch as you would mala beads, repeat your stitches to yourself. For the Mala Cowl pattern, on the knit row, repeat *bark, slip 1 yarnover* for 108 stitches. Then, on the purl row, repeat *slip 1 yarnover, burp* for 108 stitches. The barks and burps have become your mantra.

10. While repeating your mantra, keep your breath steady and easy. There's no need to force or control it. Relax your jaw. Let your thoughts float in and out without attaching to them.

11. If you find yourself getting tense trying to finish a round—perhaps you are starting to speed up or lose rhythm—stop and take a break. There is no destination here. Focus on the quality of your rhythm, not the quantity of your stitches.

12. When you have completed your meditation, close your eyes and thank yourself for your practice. Place the cowl to rest somewhere it won't be disturbed, and come back to it when you have the time to work on it peacefully to maintain a high-quality rhythm.

> ALWAYS REMIND YOURSELF OF YOUR INTENTION, AND START YOUR DEEP BREATHING WITH YOUR FEET ON THE GROUND BEFORE YOU PICK UP YOUR NEEDLES.

BEGINNINGS

STARTING ANEW EACH DAY

BKS Iyengar is the founder of Iyengar Yoga. He is recognized as one of the foremost yoga teachers in the world. In his book *Light on Life*, he writes that it should be impossible to get bored doing the same pose every day, because it's never really the same pose. The person who did the pose yesterday is a different person from the one doing it today.

Whether through my intentional actions or through forces far beyond my control, I do change each day. It's true that a slightly different me settles into Downward Dog (page 31) each time I step onto my mat or pick up my needles. That makes it easier to have a beginner's mind, to stop comparing myself to others or to my former self, and to find ease in the beauty of each moment when I am blessed with the opportunity to craft, contemplate, or move my body.

Living through cancer was a major turning point for my yoga and knitting. My yoga practice shifted from being about strength to being about rest. I suddenly felt overwhelming pain in my hands and couldn't knit for nearly as long. Even basic yoga poses became a struggle. Up to that point, my knitting and yoga practices had been progressively building. I was enjoying doing increasingly challenging poses and patterns. My vision of advancement as a rising straight line collapsed almost overnight. Knitting and yoga stopped being mountains to conquer. They became necessities just to get through my day.

> IYENGAR WRITES THAT IT SHOULD BE IMPOSSIBLE TO GET BORED DOING THE SAME POSE EVERY DAY, BECAUSE IT'S NEVER REALLY THE SAME POSE.

While I had cancer and for many years after, my yoga practice lacked movement and energy. I was usually too tired to do more than chair yoga. Even *Restorative* yoga on a mat felt like too much. I learned to modify my poses so I could continue to practice. To this day, I feel grateful for all that I learned during that time. Now I can make modifications to meet my body wherever it is in the moment.

I admit it's still a challenge for me to stop comparing the yogi I once was to the one I am now, but I work at it every day. I try to relish the five minutes I spend in Child's Pose (page 42) rather than spend that time thinking about the handstand practice I once had. I try to embrace my simple garter-stitch blanket rather than dwell on the nuances of the intarsia sweaters I used to love knitting. I welcome the experiences I am having now and give them space to teach me rather than demeaning them by comparing them to my past experiences, or to the experiences I imagine others are having. That game has no winner.

Repetition helps keep me present and encourages thoughts to exit my mind as quickly and aggressively as they sometimes enter it. Learning to be in the present moment steers me away from a pattern of negative comparisons. When I focus on where I am now rather than where I was a day ago or ten years ago, I enjoy my life as it is.

> **LEARNING TO BE IN THE PRESENT MOMENT STEERS ME AWAY FROM A PATTERN OF NEGATIVE COMPARISONS.**

BEGINNINGS

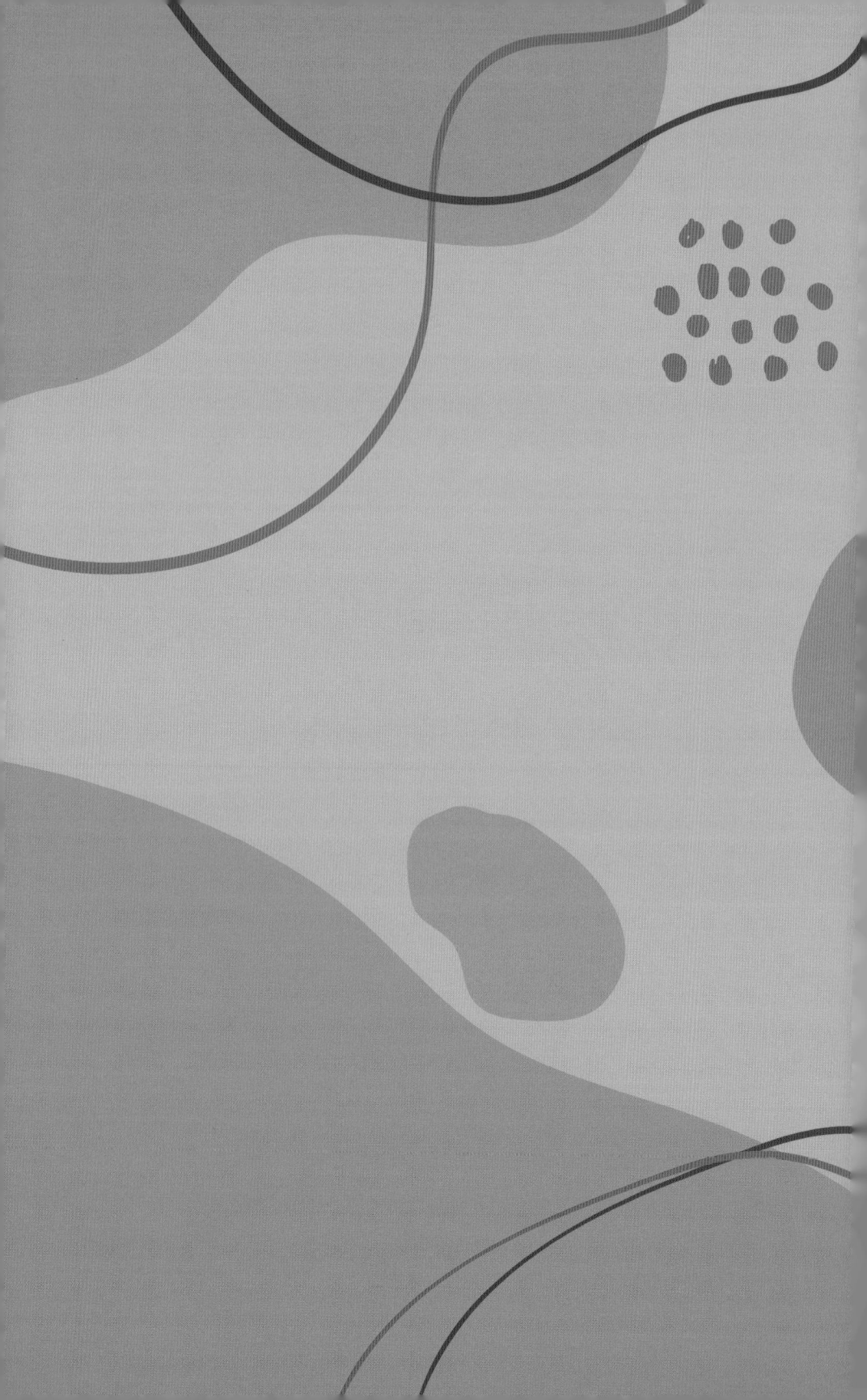

PART TWO

Contemplation

Thoughts, sensations, and emotions are nearly always flowing through our minds and bodies, even when we sleep. Because we have no choice but to live with these fluctuations, we benefit when we cultivate practices to understand and manage them, which is the focus of this chapter.

SUTRA 1.2

Yogas citta vrtti nirodhah.
Yoga is the art of quieting the mind.

WHEN WE QUIET OUR MINDS AND UNBIND OURSELVES FROM PRECONCEPTIONS, EXPECTATIONS, AND PERCEIVED LIMITATIONS, WE LIBERATE OURSELVES.

QUIETING THE MIND

When we quiet our minds and unbind ourselves from preconceptions, expectations, and perceived limitations, we liberate ourselves and open up to all sorts of new and fulfilling experiences. Quieting the mind, which we naturally do as knitters when we focus on our stitches or patterns, is the first and most important step toward growing in the direction the universe intends for us.

With a quiet mind, we can ask ourselves: How does it feel when I drop a stitch? Do I feel tension arise in my neck or jaw? When I'm confused about the instructions in a pattern, do I want to cast blame on the person who wrote it? When I resist trying a new posture or breathing technique, do I accuse the teacher of being unclear, or do I acknowledge my own fear?

When we are able to watch these thoughts and feelings without attaching ourselves to them, we can learn without judgment.

This sutra reminds us that while yoga often includes physical practice, its primary goal is to calm our inner world.

FINDING A TEACHER

Knitting and yoga are not solitary practices. Yes, we may love knitting or practicing yoga alone. And, yes, our self-discipline must come from within. But we also need guidance and support from a teacher.

Good teachers inspire and empower us. They know when to push us and when to give us space. They know how to build up our muscle memory of key skills. They show us how to become our own teachers. And they do so in a relatable way.

Yoga studios are pretty much everywhere these days, though they can differ greatly in terms of the types of yoga they offer (page 105) and their teachers' styles. Try a few studios and teachers to see what feels best.

Local knitting shops can be harder to find than yoga studios. If you don't have access to in-person instruction, the internet can be a good source as long as you find the right teacher for your learning style.

Don't be shy. Make an effort to build relationships with the people from whom you'd want to learn. It's our job to take the first step. No matter how far down the path we are, there's always someone who knows more and can inspire us with new skills.

> **GOOD TEACHERS INSPIRE AND EMPOWER US. THEY KNOW WHEN TO PUSH US AND WHEN TO GIVE US SPACE.**

CONTEMPLATION

LISTENING TO YOUR BODY

In a yoga class, our bodies are our primary teacher. Our instructors come second. They guide us, but ultimately our bodies tell us what we can and cannot do—as long as we are listening.

Listening to our bodies means knowing what is healthy for us, what will fuel us, and what can injure or deplete us. It's not about doing what we think we should do. It's about quieting the fluctuations of our mind so we can hear the body's voice. Each day our bodies have different degrees of flexibility and tension. How we stood in Mountain Pose (page 14) yesterday could be very different from today. Learning to watch for subtle changes in our equilibrium helps us feel what our bodies need most. It's all about slowing down and noticing.

All too often, if we don't listen to our bodies, we pay the price. I once took a class at a studio I was going to teach at and pushed myself too hard in my Bridge Pose, and I injured myself. As a new teacher at the studio, I felt I had something to prove. At that moment, my ego had taken over, and I wreaked havoc on my lower back. I use that memory to remind myself to listen to my body, no matter what.

These days my Ragline Knits co-conspirator, Kate, likes to joke about how when we take a yoga class together, I often end up spending most of my time lying on my mat in a *Restorative* pose. I recall a particular *Vinyasa* flow class we took in Boston after one of our Yoga + Yarn Retreats in Vermont. We had just gotten back, and I was tired from four days of teaching. After a few movements, I felt exhausted, so I got all the props I could find, set myself up in a relaxing

> LEARNING TO WATCH FOR SUBTLE CHANGES IN OUR EQUILIBRIUM HELPS US FEEL WHAT OUR BODIES NEED MOST.

58 YOGA OF YARN

position, and took a nice meditative nap. If I had pushed to follow along that day, I surely would have injured myself.

After class I felt rejuvenated and thankful that I did what my body asked. Two days later, I found out I was pregnant with my first child. My fatigue now made perfect sense. My body knew something my mind hadn't yet learned!

KNITTER'S CHOICE

We learn primarily from our own experiences.

In yoga classes most teachers offer variations for each pose, so no matter our skill level, we find something that works for us. This is called yogi's choice. Even if the teacher doesn't offer a choice, we can always ask for an adaptation. For example, if I'm taking a class and we're doing Pigeon Pose, and my knees don't feel up for it that day, I simply lie on my back with my ankle on the opposite knee. I still open my hips, but in a gentler way that works for me. The more we learn and listen to our bodies, the more easily we can identify the adjustments we need to make.

We can do the same when knitting. We often come across patterns that say something like cast on with your preferred cast-on. I call this knitter's choice. It's up to us to choose our own adventure. When we cultivate the ability to listen to the knowledge within our bodies, we encounter an array of options to choose from. For example, while making a sweater, we might add short rows for extra ease around the neck, lengthen the sleeves, or choose a special seaming technique for a refined finish.

> **THE MORE WE LEARN AND LISTEN TO OUR BODIES, THE MORE EASILY WE CAN IDENTIFY THE ADJUSTMENTS WE NEED TO MAKE.**

CONTEMPLATION

BODY SCAN

This is a 5-minute practice to help us quiet our minds, tune in, and open up to our inner knowledge. It is a great mid-knitting break. I like to set a timer, so I can close my eyes as I explore without worrying about how many minutes have passed. Read through the instructions, and make sure you understand each step before starting.

Benefits: Quiets the mind, provides feedback on how your body feels, and builds inner knowledge. Stretches the hips, lengthens the spine, and relieves stiffness in the neck. **Props:** Chair, timer

If you have back pain or high or low blood pressure, avoid this posture.

1. Sit in a chair with your legs bent and feet hip distance apart. Set a timer for 5 minutes.
2. If there is a table in front of you, stack your forearms on top of each other and rest your forehead on your arms. Elongate your spine.
3. If there's no table, take your hands to your knees and, with care, lower your upper body between your legs. Let your arms hang toward the floor. Let your head relax down toward the floor with your shoulders moving away from your ears.
4. Once you feel steady, close your eyes and bring focus to your feet. Notice how they are pressing into the floor. See if you can feel the entire sole of each foot on the ground. Lift and wiggle your toes. Then place them back down on the ground.

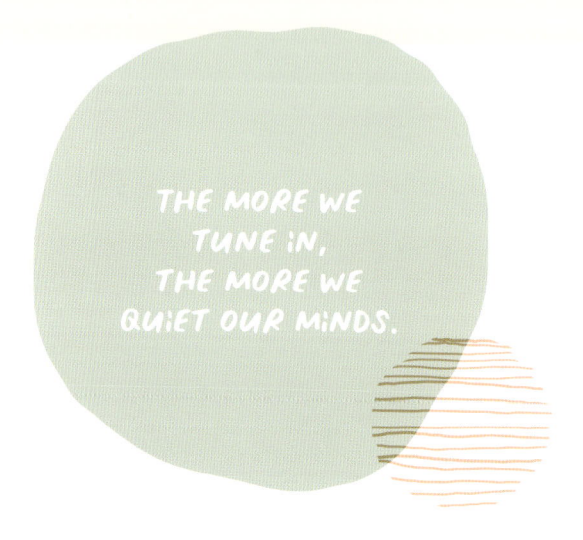

> THE MORE WE TUNE IN, THE MORE WE QUIET OUR MINDS.

5. Bring your awareness to each part of your body. Start from your toes and work your way up to the top of your head. There is no rush as you move up your body. During the scan, reflect on what you notice about each part of your body. If your mind wanders, coax yourself to focus on your breath for a few moments, then return to scanning your body.

   Notice how your breath is flowing. Do you notice any sensations like tingling, tightness, warmth, pulsing, coolness? Are there any judgments or powerful emotions entering your mind?

6. Notice without judgment when the mind wanders. Acknowledge it and return to the sensations in your body.

7. After you have scanned each individual body part, feel your body as a single, pulsating entity. Ask yourself these questions.
   - What do I notice?
   - What is my body telling me?
   - Am I thinking about what I believe I should be feeling right now?
   - Am I being true to the present moment?

8. Try not to judge yourself if you feel like you're not doing this right. There is no right or wrong way to do a body scan. The mind will wander. You don't need to make changes to your body. Tune in to what's happening.

9. When your alarm goes off, don't rush away. Wiggle your body gently and transition back into your day with ease.

SUPPORTED PIGEON POSE

Pigeon Pose, *kapotasana*, is a deep hip opener that a lot of people like, but it can be challenging on the knees. That's why I like to teach Supported Pigeon Pose, *salamba eka pada rajakapotasana*, a version where we use a chair to support the body and give our tight hips a chance to open while keeping the knees safe.

Benefits: Opens the inner and outer hips. **Props**: Chair, blanket

If you have low back pain or hip or knee injury, avoid this posture.

1. Stand facing the chair, with the seat of the chair closest to you. Place a folded blanket on the seat of the chair. Bend forward and place your hands on the back of the chair.
2. Bring your right knee to the back right corner of the seat.
3. Gently place your right foot off the near left edge of the seat, flexing the ankle to protect the delicate knee joint.
4. Straighten the left leg. Tuck the back toes under for a more active stretch. Or, for a more restorative position, point the toes and rest the top of the foot on the floor.

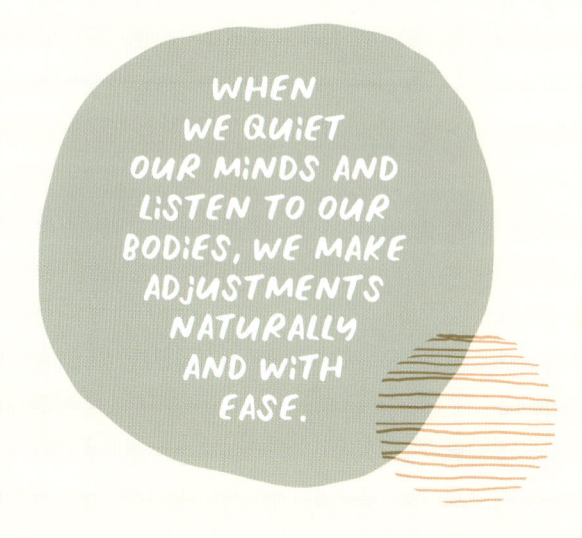

> WHEN WE QUIET OUR MINDS AND LISTEN TO OUR BODIES, WE MAKE ADJUSTMENTS NATURALLY AND WITH EASE.

5. Rest your forearms on the back of the chair and lower your forehead to your arms. Take 10 to 20 deep breaths.
6. With care, lift your head and press your hands into the back of the chair to rise back up to standing. Bend forward and place your hands on the back of the chair.
7. Bring your left knee to the back left corner of the seat.
8. Gently place your left foot off the near right edge of the seat, flexing the ankle to protect the delicate knee joint.
9. Straighten the right leg. Tuck the back toes under for a more active stretch. Or, for a more restorative position, point the toes and rest the top of the foot on the floor.
10. Rest your forearms on the back of the chair and lower your forehead to your arms. Take 10 to 20 deep breaths.
11. With care, lift your head and press your hands into the back of the chair to rise back up to standing.

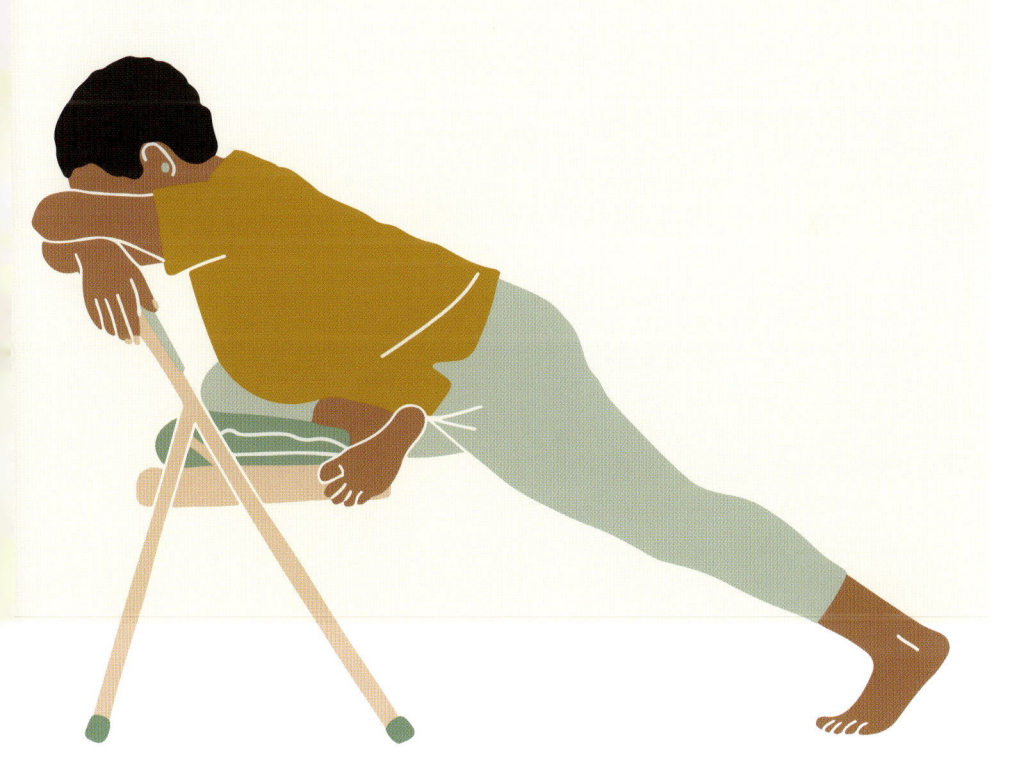

> FINDING OUR EDGE AS KNITTERS MEANS TRYING NEW STITCH PATTERNS OR MORE COMPLICATED PROJECTS OUTSIDE OUR COMFORT ZONE.

FINDING AND EXPLORING OUR EDGE

Finding our edge during a yoga class means challenging ourselves to the point of learning something new without going too far and building up resistance or risking injury. When we hold a yoga pose a little longer than usual, we might start to wobble or our muscles might shake. The mind will begin telling us to back off, but if we can pause and stay in the moment with controlled breathing—if we can find some comfort within the discomfort—we will find our edge. If our breathing loses its rhythm, it's time to gently back off.

Finding our edge as knitters means trying new stitch patterns or more complicated projects outside our comfort zone. If we only know a knit stitch, then our edge might be a purl or trying short rows for the first time. If we love mosaic knitting but have always been intimidated by working with colors, then that might be our edge.

Some days learning a new skill feels like a chore, and we feel ourselves resisting it, often without even knowing why. We stick to what we know. But some days the resistance isn't there. It's our job to notice that absence of resistance and seize the opportunity to explore it. When we explore our edge, we naturally turn inward and are able to watch our thought patterns and bodily sensations.

With a quiet mind, see what questions and ideas arise. The key is to watch these reactions and responses to our discomfort without attaching ourselves to them. We can learn without judgment. We can be comfortable in an uncomfortable situation.

THE POWER OF SILENCE

Knitting lends itself to quiet and contemplation. Embrace these beautiful gifts. Every once in a while, curl up in a favorite chair, couch, cushion, or corner of the floor, and agree to just be with your knitting. Just knitting. In silence, the sounds around us amplify. We hear our own breathing. We notice the click of our knitting needles. Over time, our focus turns inward. When we do this, we meditate, whether we choose to call it meditation or not.

During my yoga teacher and yoga therapy training, I was sometimes required to spend entire days in silence. I was expected to go about my regular routine without uttering a word. These challenging, powerful experiences called my attention to how much excessive, unnecessary talking happens over the course of a day.

It takes patience and practice to be with ourselves in silence. When we invite our thoughts to flow in, and then flow out as easily as they entered, we learn to hear what we are really saying to ourselves internally without reacting to it. We foster a sense of ease when we sit and knit in silence. If we feel restless, we bring our minds back to tracking our stitch patterns. We do this until we outlast the restlessness, learning a little bit more about ourselves with each passing moment. In silence, truth finds us.

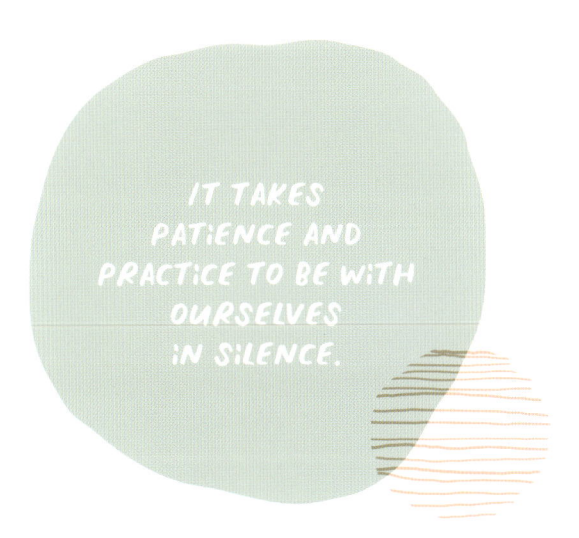

> IN SILENCE, TRUTH FINDS US.

> IT TAKES PATIENCE AND PRACTICE TO BE WITH OURSELVES IN SILENCE.

CONTEMPLATION

FOLLOWING INTUITION

Intuition is our ability to understand or know something immediately without overthinking it. Sometimes we don't even know it in our heads—we know it in our bones, our heart, our gut, or our cells. This makes it extremely personal. We can't possibly understand all the consequences of our decisions before we make them. Instead, we trust that if we follow our intuition, then we have made the right decision regardless of the outcome.

> SOMETIMES WE DON'T EVEN KNOW IT IN OUR HEADS— WE KNOW IT IN OUR BONES, OUR HEART, OUR GUT, OR OUR CELLS.

I like to think of myself as an intuitive knitter. When I'm designing a new project, I'll usually follow my gut first and do the math later. Rather than applying a formula, I'll cast on the number of stitches that feels right based on past experience. Even if I'm off, I've seized an opportunity to hone my intuition. Of course, this only works if I'm making something for myself. If I'm planning to write a pattern to publish or share with a friend, I'm a bit more methodical from the start. I don't want anyone else to suffer if my intuition gets it wrong!

Daily meditations, breathing exercises, and moments of silence clear our minds and open us to the possibility of listening to our inner guidance. We all have intuition, but some of us are more tuned into it than others. Yoga and knitting cultivate our intuition and keep us connected to it. So, let's practice some intuitive knitting and have some fun with it.

CULTIVATING INTUITION

Intuition comes naturally to some people. For others it is a skill to be learned, one that becomes a natural habit with practice. Try this short exercise to cultivate your intuition.

Benefits: Cultivates intuition and self-knowledge. **Props:** None

1. Find a comfortable place to sit, stand, or lie on the floor.
2. Breathe in and say *inhale* to yourself. Breathe out and say *exhale* to yourself. Repeat 5 times.
3. Check in with your body. What sensations, thoughts, or emotions do you notice? Continue noticing what you feel for 10 more breaths.
4. Now ask yourself, *What do I need right now?* Take note of whatever your first reaction is to that question.
5. What smells and sounds do you notice? Take note of whatever your first reaction is to that question.
6. Place your hands on your heart center and offer love to yourself. Breathe steadily in this position for a few moments.

Repeat this practice periodically to cultivate your intuition. The more you practice, the more likely your intuition will be active when you need it.

> DAILY MEDITATIONS, BREATHING EXERCISES, AND MOMENTS OF SILENCE CLEAR OUR MINDS AND OPEN US TO THE POSSIBILITY OF LISTENING TO OUR INNER GUIDANCE.

INTUITIVE KNITTING

The art of intuitive knitting is listening to your gut—or your bones, heart, cells, or anywhere your body stores knowledge that communicates in a different way from the knowledge stored in the prefrontal cortex, the part of the brain responsible for our intentional reasoning and conscious decisions.

When we use our intuition to pick the next knitting project, we create a deep sense of connection. We take ownership over our project in our bodies and not merely in our heads. The knowledge stored in our bodies can continue to help us all the way to the finished item.

Let's say you've found a gorgeous new skein of yarn at your local shop. Your body already knows you're going to buy it before your brain does. Okay, that's a wonderful feeling, but what now? How do you decide what to knit? Maybe the people at the shop have some good ideas. Maybe you've looked online to gain some inspiration. But maybe this time you want to try something new or explore beyond your comfort zone.

Benefits: Cultivates intuition and builds a foundation for advanced knitting practices. **Props:** Chair, table, yarn, needles, pen, paper

1. PREPARE: Gather your supplies and sit down at a table, preferably a favorite spot at home or outside if it's a nice day.

2. QUERY: Hold the yarn in your hands and gently ask yourself what you want to knit.

3. BREATHE: With your yarn still in your hands, close your eyes. Inhale, filling your lungs and allowing your abdomen to expand to its fullest. When you feel like you can't fit any more air in your belly, exhale out through your mouth until all the air is released. Repeat this breath for a few more rounds. While you do, keep a gentle hold on your yarn throughout. You might try moving your fingers up and down the strands. Feel the fibers as they caress your hands. Relax your tongue away from the roof of your mouth. As you breathe in through your nose, see if you can sense where the breath is flowing throughout your body. Can you feel expansion across the entire body as you inhale and a full release as you exhale?

4. DRAW: After your last exhale, open your eyes and draw a rough sketch of something you could imagine knitting. Don't hesitate or judge, just do it. Bear in mind that when I do this exercise, what I draw looks like my preschooler's artwork. How it looks does not matter. The goal is to have fun.

5. COUNT: If you're still not interested in drawing or you find yourself getting frustrated, put down your pen! Pick up your yarn again and begin counting your breaths. Inhale, counting slowly from 1 to 4, and then exhale, counting slowly from 1 to 5. Continue like this for 2 minutes, focusing on the numbers and the luscious yarn in your fingers.

6. KNIT: Pick up your needles, cast on 20 stitches, and knit. Make a garter-stitch swatch to start. As you're knitting, the yarn will take shape, and you will see what it needs—maybe a little stockinette stitch, ribbing, or a few yarnovers. Play with it and see what it becomes.

7. PATTERN: Once you have a small swatch, at least 4 inches (10 cm) long, you may have a better idea of what you want it to become. The yarn comes alive as you knit it and it expresses its own energy. Design your pattern from your swatch and start writing. If you don't have a final pattern in mind or aren't comfortable writing your own patterns (yet!), go online and explore patterns similar to your swatch and ideas. Take your time and see if you can make a choice that resonates in your gut, not your head.

> TO OPEN UP YOUR CHANNELS OF INTUITION, TRY THE CULTIVATING INTUITION PRACTICE (PAGE 67) FIRST, THEN COME BACK TO THIS ONE.

KNITTER'S EIGHT-FOLD PATH

The Eight-Fold Path is a yogi's journey to living a purposeful life, an outline for moral and ethical conduct, self-discipline, attention to one's health, and spiritual growth. It is a lesson in how the whole is both greater than and different from the sum of its constituent parts. Many yogis have spent their lives on the journey of the Eight-Fold Path. Let's just say it ain't easy! But perhaps we can achieve a kind of Eight-Fold Path in our knitting, and maybe over time that translates to other parts of our lives, too.

What I call the Knitter's Eight-Fold Path marries the contentment and purpose we radiate when we combine mastering knitting techniques with valuing yarn and its origins, caring for and sharing finished knits, and contributing to a community of fellow knitters. These are distinct goals, and all of them are required to achieve the Knitter's Eight-Fold Path. The journey we take on this path can ease the anxiety and fear at the core of our human experience.

SUTRA 2.29

Yama niyama asana pranayama pratyahara dharana dhyana samadhi astau angani.

yama	niyama	asana	pranayama
abstinence	observance	posture practice	breath control

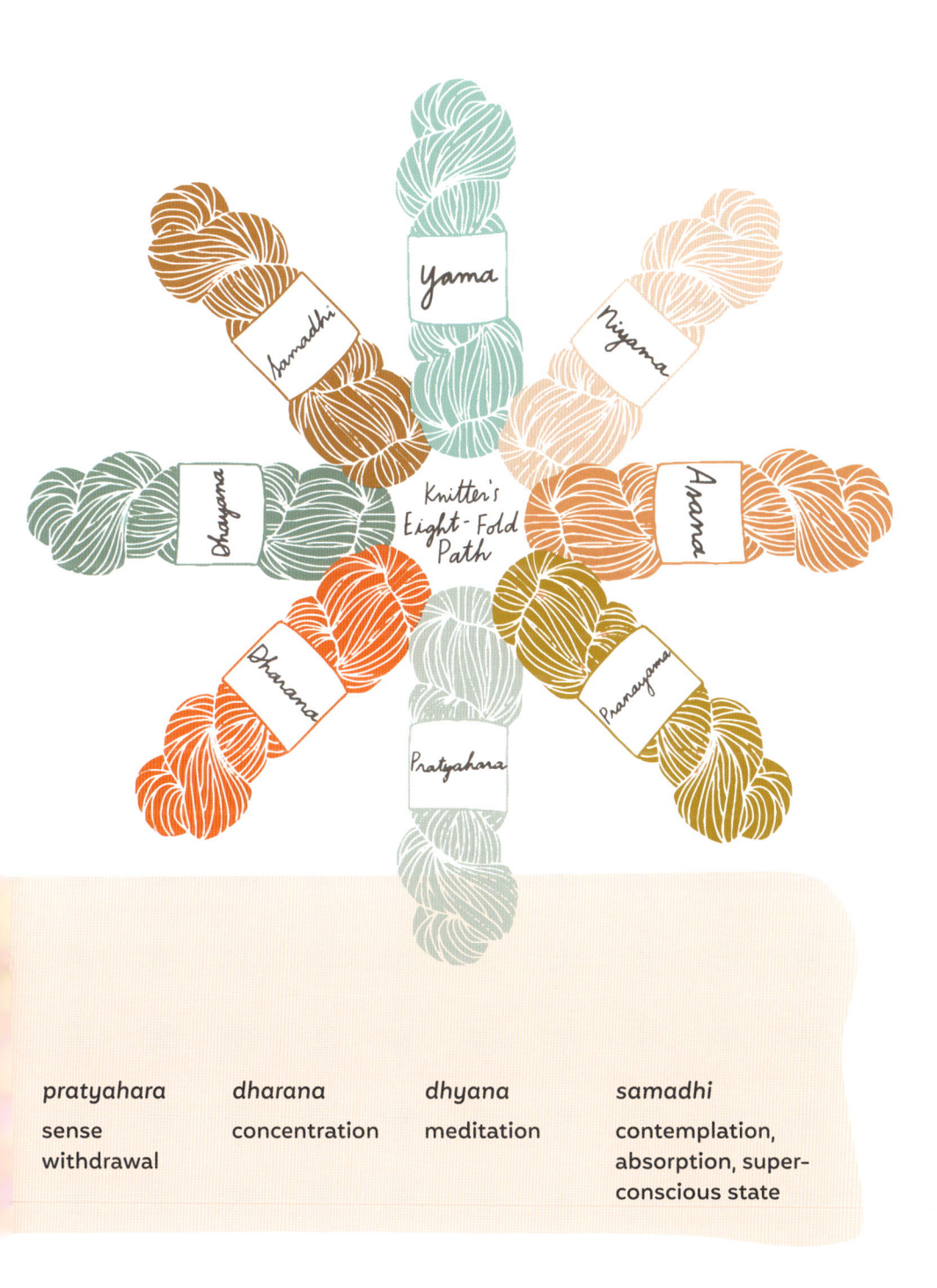

Knitter's Eight-Fold Path

- Yama
- Niyama
- Asana
- Pranayama
- Pratyahara
- Dharana
- Dhyana
- Samadhi

pratyahara	dharana	dhyana	samadhi
sense withdrawal	concentration	meditation	contemplation, absorption, super-conscious state

CONTEMPLATION

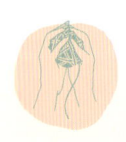

KNITTER'S EIGHT-FOLD PATH

Eight-Fold Path	Yoga Interpretation
Yama	Ethical considerations, the rules we follow and the restraint we show to live in harmony with other humans.
ahimsa	*Ahimsa* means nonviolence, being kind to ourselves and to others. This includes not causing physical harm to ourselves or others and preventing emotional injury as well.
satya	*Satya* means truth, or not lying. It asks us to live in a way that honors our highest truth. When we practice *satya*, we are honest with ourselves and others, and we refrain from judgment. We act and speak with intention.
asteya	*Asteya* means nonstealing, a moral principle for all humans to follow.
brahmacharya	*Brahmacharya* is the practice of energy conservation and moderation. It teaches us to focus our energy and spend time on what fuels us rather than what depletes us.
aparigraha	*Aparigraha* means nonhoarding or nonattachment. A practicing yogi does not try to grasp or cling to all things material.

Knitting Interpretation

Rules of conduct for interacting with and morally supporting fellow knitters.

We consider where our wool comes from and the local communities it supports, the shearing process, and the treatment of animals.

We are honest with ourselves and our fellow knitters. We speak our truth in a manner that builds positive ties with all those in our knitting community.

We don't photocopy knitting patterns or otherwise avoid paying for a pattern we want to try. We don't overuse or rely on someone else's resources to their detriment. We don't take advantage of the generosity of others.

We prioritize our projects and foster relationships that are important to us. We knit with intention, and we direct our energy to that purpose when we knit.

We use our yarn, needles, and stash without hoarding. We share our supplies and do not cling to them unnecessarily.

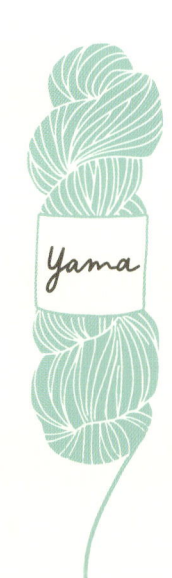

(continued on next page)

KNITTER'S EIGHT-FOLD PATH (continued from previous page)

Eight-Fold Path	Yoga Interpretation
Niyama	Self-disciplines representing how we care for ourselves.
shaucha	*Shaucha* means cleanliness as a way of taking care of our body and mind. We take a shower not only to clean the body, but also to clear the mind and reset our thought patterns.
santosha	*Santosha* means contentment, being satisfied with what we have. Because the world is ever-changing, we find our peace within.
tapas	*Tapas* means self-discipline. The main way we practice *tapas* is through dedication to our craft through continual practice. Showing up and doing the work requires consistent repetition and discipline. We are better able to do this when we meditate and quiet our mind.
svadhyaya	*Svadhyaya* is the examination of our self and spirituality, often through the study of spiritual books. It emphasizes our commitment to growth.
isvara pranidhana	*Isvara pranidhana* means surrender. When we allow ourselves to believe in a power greater than ourselves and look beyond ourselves, we start to experience change from within. A deep peace enters us when we realize that we are here to serve that greater power, and we can trust the universe to support us.

Knitting Interpretation

Rules of conduct we follow as knitters. This includes how we care for our yarn, needles, and notions, how we block or finish our knits, and how we start a new project with the aim of caring for ourselves.

We keep our yarn, needles, and other supplies in good shape so they will serve their purpose in supporting our knitting for a long time to come.

Contentment reminds us to focus on the knitting project in our hands. It also expresses the concept of loving and accepting imperfections, as nothing in life is permanent.

Even when our stitches fall off our needles, or our sweater felts in the wash, we keep going because we accept our mistakes as equally as our successes. Daily repetition is the foundation of our growth.

We read knitting patterns, books, magazines, and essays to promote our growth and knowledge of ourselves as knitters.

We cast on for our next project with faith and peace that what will happen is what should happen, whatever that may be.

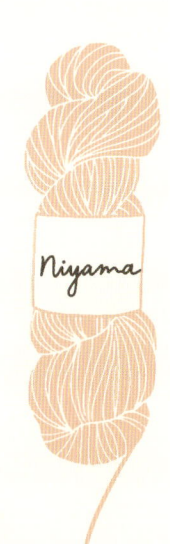

(continued on next page)

KNITTER'S EIGHT-FOLD PATH *(continued from previous page)*

Eight-Fold Path	Yoga Interpretation
Asana	Physical postures.
Pranayama	*Pranayama* is regulation of our breath. Yogis believe the more we extend our breath, the longer we live. Different breathing techniques can create an internal sense of calm or create more energy within our bodies.
Pratyahara	*Pratyahara* is sense withdrawal. Through the practice of withdrawing our attention from external influences, we achieve greater ease within. The idea is to learn to connect with the inner world so that eventually we enter a super-conscious state.
Dharana	*Dharana* is concentration. When the mind can focus its undivided attention on the present moment, we experience *dharana*.
Dhyana	*Dhyana* is often translated as meditation. *Dhyana* is the evolution of the mind from automatic responses to a state of heightened awareness.
Samadhi	*Samadhi* means intense concentration, or a hyper-conscious state achieved through meditation. This is often considered the state of enlightenment reached through fully absorbed contemplation.

Knitting Interpretation

We take care of our body through yoga movements so that we are able to knit for a long time to come.

We engage in breathing practices to enhance our knitting experience. Our breath can ignite warmth or cool us down and create a greater sense of calm.

The less distracted we are by sounds or other elements around us as we knit, the more our internal sensors can tune in. We find the external world disturbs us less. While knitting, try closing your eyes or putting on noise-canceling headphones.

We experience *dharana* when our mind, body, and stitches are all riding the same wavelength without our thoughts getting in the way.

We experience *dhyana* when we reach an elevated awareness of each moment while knitting. We are not on autopilot, mindlessly knitting and purling. Instead, we are fully conscious, without attachment.

As knitters we might reach a high level of intense concentration when we are working with four colors and with both hands all at the same time, only occasionally needing to glance at the chart. While this is not enlightenment, it is a good example of a knitter headed toward a super-conscious state.

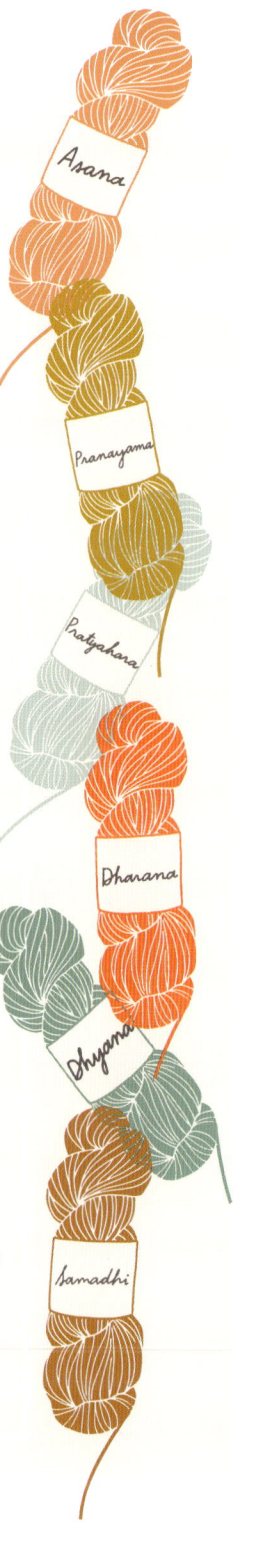

OPPOSITE THOUGHTS

There is a concept in yoga called *pratipaksha bhavana* that teaches us how to move past our negative thoughts. The gist is simple: When we notice negative thoughts squatting in our brains, we send in opposite or positive thoughts. Pessimistic or unproductive thoughts can prevent us from finding peace or enjoying our knitting and yoga.

By cultivating a positive or compassionate thought each time a negative or judgmental one arises, we rewire our thinking. If we do this often enough, we can train ourselves to start from that positive space, and we don't need to replace our negative thoughts anymore.

So, let's put *pratipaksha bhavana* to work for us in our knitting today. This practice changes our outlook from cynical to compassionate so that we can feel inspired, hopeful, and motivated. It may not heal our hurting hands or cure other ailments or worries, but we might notice that those sore body parts don't aggravate us quite as much when we have a sunnier disposition.

SUTRA 2.33

Vitarka badhane pratipaksha bhavanam.

When disturbed by negative thoughts, opposite (positive) ones should be thought of.

REWIRING

Sometimes when we're knitting, we get confused about what we're doing and blame it on our perceived inadequacy. Next time this happens try telling yourself *I'm an amazing knitter*, and *I can do this*. If you find it's too challenging to rewire from negative to positive thoughts this way, try placing yourself in a nurturing environment. For example, ask your best knitter friend to remind you of your wonderful abilities. The more often you are able to replace detrimental thoughts with affirmative ones, the sooner your mind will rewire itself. This exercise will help you with the rewiring.

Benefits: Rewires the mind and cultivates a disposition that readies us for whatever life may send our way. **Props:** Yarn, needles, knitting project, timer

1. Note the time or start the stopwatch feature on your timer and start knitting.
2. Pay attention to where your mind goes while you knit. Are your thoughts focused on the stitches or on something else? When a thought enters your mind, note if it is negative or positive. A negative thought is usually one that has a built-in expectation that isn't being met. Identify that expectation without judgment.
3. Note how much time has elapsed from when you started knitting to your first negative thought.
4. Once you identify the negative thought, think of the exact opposite self-affirming thought. Say it to yourself or, even better, out loud. Repeat this each time a negative thought arises.
5. Take a break from knitting every 20 minutes. Your break can be 30 seconds or 5 minutes, but be sure to shake out your hands and remain conscious of the thoughts popping into your mind. Continue to counter the judgmental thoughts with compassionate ones.

Do this practice daily and keep track of how long you knit until your first negative thought arises. If you practice often enough, the time it takes for your first unproductive thought to arise will increase significantly in a matter of weeks!

LOVING-KINDNESS

A yoga teacher once explained to me that we don't have to like everyone, but we do have to love everyone. When I first heard this, I wasn't convinced. But I trusted and respected her, so I took her words to heart and tried my best to offer my love all around. My attempts were far from perfect and often misguided. But sincerely trying to love even the people I didn't like helped me understand what she meant. I began to see that focusing on what I didn't like about other people was no different than taking poison and expecting them to get sick. I was the one suffering, not them. When I relieved myself of the burden that disliking them placed on me, I felt a kind of freedom that made me giddy. And I came to a deeper understanding: As we cultivate the ability to express loving-kindness toward ourselves and others, the power of those feelings begins to emanate to everyone around us.

Today I love to practice and share a Buddhist meditation method that fosters a direct connection with the love my yoga teacher was talking about. This type of meditation is called loving-kindness, or *metta bhavana*. On page 82 I offer a knitter's variation of this practice.

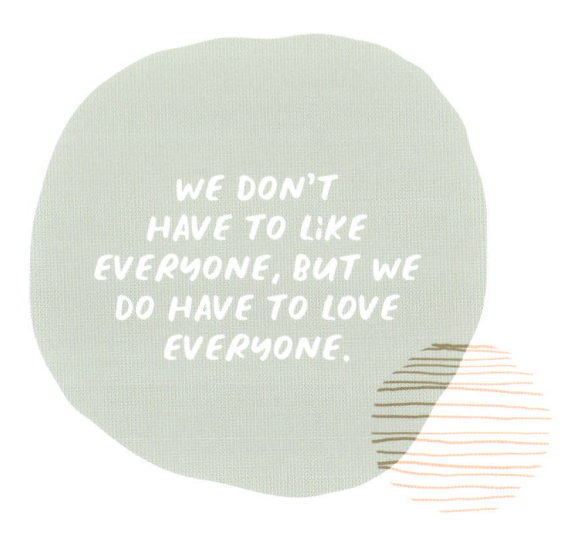

> WE DON'T HAVE TO LIKE EVERYONE, BUT WE DO HAVE TO LOVE EVERYONE.

Many knitters practice loving-kindness naturally without even knowing it. Every time we knit an item for a loved one, a charity, a cancer patient, or a friend of a friend, we are practicing loving-kindness. When we choose to practice developing compassion, we reduce stress and boost our overall well-being. Of course, we can offer love toward ourselves, loved ones, and friends. But can we do it consistently, even when it's hard? Even when we feel burnt out? Even toward someone who has wronged us? It can be tough to wish loving-kindness when we're in conflict with someone, or when we're too tired even to think. This is why the meditation starts with showing grace to ourselves, our loved ones, and our friends. It's a warmup to the hard stuff.

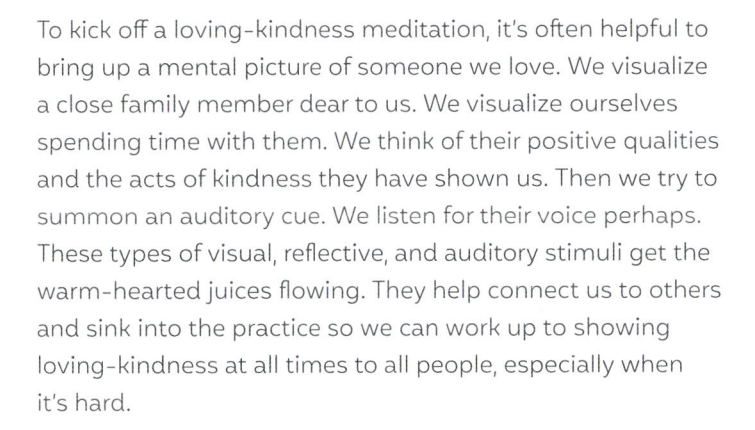

To kick off a loving-kindness meditation, it's often helpful to bring up a mental picture of someone we love. We visualize a close family member dear to us. We visualize ourselves spending time with them. We think of their positive qualities and the acts of kindness they have shown us. Then we try to summon an auditory cue. We listen for their voice perhaps. These types of visual, reflective, and auditory stimuli get the warm-hearted juices flowing. They help connect us to others and sink into the practice so we can work up to showing loving-kindness at all times to all people, especially when it's hard.

WHEN WE CHOOSE TO PRACTICE LOVING-KINDNESS, WE REDUCE STRESS AND BOOST OUR OVERALL WELL-BEING.

LOVING-KINDNESS MEDITATION

This is a variation on a traditional loving-kindness meditation. When first starting out, pick an easy project—perhaps a garter-stitch scarf.

Benefits: Rewires the mind and cultivates a disposition that readies us for whatever life may send our way. **Props:** Easy knitting project, needles, chair or blankets

1. Sit in a chair with your back supported and feet planted on the ground. Or sit on blankets on the floor in Easy Pose (page 12).

2. Once in a supported position, take a few deep inhales and long exhales. For a few minutes, feel or imagine your breath moving through the center of your chest around your heart. Knit a few stitches as you breathe deeply.

3. As you continue to knit, start offering love to yourself. Repeat slowly and steadily: *May I be happy. May I be well. May I be safe. May I be peaceful and at ease.* Allow yourself to sink into these intentions. Loving-kindness meditation is about connecting to the intention of wishing yourself and others happiness. If feelings of warmth, friendliness, or love arise in the body or mind, connect to them, and allow them to grow as you repeat the phrases. Continue knitting and breathing gently as the stitches and offerings of love expand.

4. Summon an image of someone in your life who has deeply cared for you. Hold this image in your mind's eye. As you knit, repeat: *May [name] be happy. May [name] be well. May [name] be safe. May [name] be peaceful and at ease.*

5. Allow your love for this person to go into your knitting project. As feelings of loving-kindness arise, connect them with the phrases so the feelings increase as you repeat the words. Breath by breath, stitch by stitch, offer kindness to the world.

6. Now recall someone you don't really know—a person who doesn't conjure positive or negative feelings. Stick with the first person that comes to mind. Don't overthink it. Hold an image of the neutral person in your mind's eye to reinforce the intentions expressed in the phrases. Notice if you find focusing a challenge. You may feel bored, or your thoughts may have bounced elsewhere. Simply note if that happens.

7. Still knitting, repeat the phrases: *May [name] be happy. May [name] be well. May [name] be safe. May [name] be peaceful and at ease.*

8. Now think of a person who gives you difficulty. Hold an image of them in your mind's eye to reinforce the intentions expressed in the phrases. With each stitch, repeat phrases of loving-kindness toward them: *May [name] be happy. May [name] be well. May [name] be safe. May [name] be peaceful and at ease.*

9. If more than one difficult person popped into your mind, slowly repeat this step for each of them. Notice if feelings like anger, grief, or sadness arise. These are signs that your heart is softening and revealing what it holds inside. Direct loving-kindness toward these feelings. If that feels challenging, switch to noticing the feelings as they happen. Above all, do not judge yourself. Let your feelings come out freely without getting in their way.

10. Finish the meditation by offering loving-kindness to all living beings in the world: *May all beings be happy. May all beings be well. May all beings be safe. May all beings be peaceful and at ease.*

11. Deepen your breath and place your project off to the side. Stand and stretch a little. Allow the feelings of happiness and peace to settle into your body, mind, and spirit.

Repeat each time you pick up this knitting project.

LOVING-KINDNESS ON-THE-GO

You don't have to limit the loving-kindness meditation to quiet times at home. When you're out running errands, shopping for yarn, or sitting in traffic, you can repeat the mantra: *May all beings be happy, may all beings be well, may all beings be safe, may all beings be peaceful and at ease.* You can take this practice with you wherever you go.

SINGLE-POINTED FOCUS

A consistent single-pointed focus gives us the superpower of remaining present with one task when life, other people, or even our own senses pull us in many directions. Being able to summon a single-pointed focus when we most need it reduces stress and calms the mind and body.

We develop single-pointed focus by training our *drishti*, or gaze (page 32). Centering the mind's eye on a candle flame—called candle gazing, or *tratak*—is often a good starting point to develop our *drishti*. Because I don't have candles all over my house, I usually modify this meditation from focusing on a candle flame to focusing on my knitting needles, which somehow seem to be strewn everywhere!

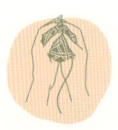

> BEING ABLE TO SUMMON A SINGLE-POINTED FOCUS WHEN WE MOST NEED IT REDUCES STRESS AND CALMS THE MIND AND BODY.

NEEDLE CONCENTRATION

Focusing our *drishti* on our knitting needles trains us to concentrate, strengthening our meditation practice.

Benefits: Reduces stress and anxiety, and develops concentration.
Props: Chair or 2 blankets, knitting project with simple stitch pattern, timer

1. Gather your project and seat yourself either on a chair or on the floor on 2 blankets in Easy Pose (page 12). Set a timer for 5 to 10 minutes.
2. Maintain a comfortable neck position with your chin parallel to the floor. With a soft gaze, look down at your needles.
3. Focus your gaze on the tip of the working needle as it maneuvers into the stitch.
4. With your attention focused on that point, allow the breath to flow in and out through your nose.
5. Thoughts will arise, and you may feel compelled to move your body. Try to resist engaging in the thoughts, and only move the hands as you knit.
6. Your eyes will want to wander to other points in the room, or even to the yarn. As best you can, keep your eyes on the movements of the needles.
7. When the timer goes off, put your knitting down and close your eyes. Offer gratitude to yourself for taking the time to meditate.

RESTING OUR EYES

When we knit, read, and watch screens, our eyes are working hard.

Performing a few eye exercises between knitting sessions helps to reduce stress on the eyes.

EYE YOGA

I recommend doing this sequence after knitting for an extended period of time or whenever else you feel you need it.

Benefits: Reduces stress on eyes, produces natural moisture to cleanse eyes, and improves concentration. **Prop:** Timer

If you have an eye injury, avoid this practice.

1. BLINKING GAZE PRACTICE: Set a timer for 2 minutes. Lift your chin parallel to the floor. Blink for 4 seconds, then close your eyes and rest for 4 seconds. Repeat until the timer goes off.
2. EYE ROLLS: Look up, right, down, and left. Repeat the same rotation smoothly, rolling the eyes at a slow pace in each direction.
3. Repeat the eye rolls a total of 3 times, then gaze in front of you for 10 seconds.
4. Blink 10 times in a row.
5. Repeat Steps 1-4, rotating your eyes in the opposite direction (up, left, down right).
6. Set the timer for 2 minutes. Lift your chin parallel to the floor. Close your eyes and look into the backs of your eyelids until the timer goes off.
7. Place the base of the palms of your hands gently against your eyelids, and take 3 breaths before releasing your hands and fluttering your eyes open.

Eye Pillow

Use this eye pillow to promote your relaxation response. Place it over your eyes and let it block out light and calm your nervous system, ideally for at least 5 minutes every day.

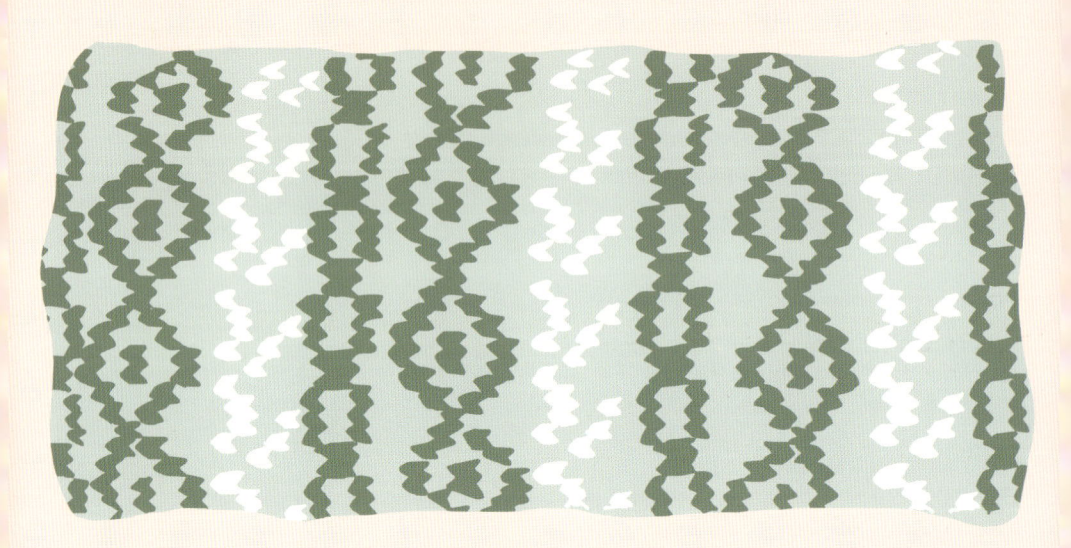

Size & Dimensions
4.5" (11 cm) wide by 9" (23 cm) long

Materials
DK weight yarn. Choose something that will feel good on the face (such as a silk, linen, or cotton blend).

Yarn A: 75 yards (69 meters)

Yarn B: 30 yards (28 meters)

Yarn C: 15 yards (14 meters)

Size US 5 (3.75 mm) double-pointed needles, or size needed to obtain gauge.

Scrap yarn for provisional cast-on, stitch marker, tapestry needle

¾ cup dried beans

½ cup dried rice or orzo

½ cup dried lavender

2-3 drops lavender essential oil

Be sure to consider the user's scent preferences or allergies. You can always swap the essential oil and skip the dried lavender.

25 stitches and 26 rounds = 4" (10 cm) in Eye Pillow Pattern from chart, after blocking.

Always use a needle size that will result in the correct gauge after blocking.

Pillow

Cast on 60 stitches using scrap yarn and provisional cast-on; distribute stitches evenly onto 3 or 4 double-pointed needles. Join in round, being careful not to twist stitches. Place marker at beginning of round.

Begin Eye Pillow Motif from chart; work Rounds 1–19 a total of 3 times, then Rounds 1–4 once more. Piece should measure 9.5" (24 cm) from cast-on edge. Cut yarns B and C.

Place 30 stitches onto each of 2 double-pointed needles; with WSs together (seam will be on the outside), using yarn A and Three-Needle Bind-Off, bind off all stitches.

Block the piece to measurements. Allow to air-dry completely.

Combine the filling ingredients in a bowl. Transfer to pillow once it is dry.

Place the live stitches from the provisional cast-on onto 2 double-pointed needles; with WSs together, using yarn A and Three-Needle Bind-Off, bind off all stitches. Weave in the ends and enjoy!

Eye Pillow Motif

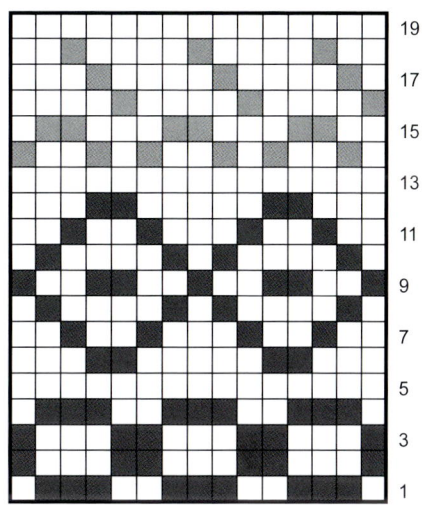

☐ Yarn A
■ Yarn B
▨ Yarn C

Time to Relax

I suggest turning on calming instrumental music and lying down somewhere super-comfy. If you want to make sure eye makeup doesn't rub off on your pillow, lay a tissue over your eyes and place the pillow on top. Relax with the pillow over your eyes for at least 5 minutes. Repeat a soothing mantra to bring your mind back to center if you notice your mind wandering places that don't serve you.

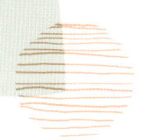

MAKING SPACE

Cables create texture, draw the eye in, and make even a non-knitter appreciate both the difficulty and magic of knitting. Sure, we can spend ages making complicated cables that turn left, right, and every which way. But an easy cable can also be striking.

EAGLE ARMS POSE

One of my favorite ways to find space in my upper body—and to remind myself to create space everywhere in my life—is Eagle Arms Pose, *garudasana*, where we wrap our forearms around each other. I liken this posture to a cable stitch because the quality of the twist depends upon our ability to create space to combat compression.

Try Eagle Pose right before you start knitting and right after you finish.

Benefits: Builds confidence and releases tension in the neck, shoulders, and upper back between the shoulder blades. **Prop:** Chair (optional)

If you have neck or shoulder pain, avoid this posture.

1. Sit in a chair with your feet planted on the ground. If you've already been sitting for a while, try standing.

2. Shake your hands like you are drying them off. Do a few gentle neck rolls and then roll your shoulders back. Don't forget to breathe; notice your inhales and exhales. Maintain a steady, even breath throughout this posture.

3. Stretch your arms out to the sides at shoulder level. Then bring your arms in front of you, and cross the right arm over the left. Place the palms of your hands on your back, and walk your hands toward each other along your shoulder blades.

4. Squeeze, giving yourself a big hug. You can stay right here as you release your shoulders away from your ears. Hold for 5 long inhales and exhales.

5. When you're ready for more, release the hug, but keep your elbows together at chest height. Wrap your forearms around each other so they are intertwined and your palms come together. If that isn't happening as planned, keep the elbows interlocked and the backs of the forearms pressed together.

When knitting cables, we compress the fabric unless we add spacer stitches. Our bodies benefit from spacer stitches too, so we can prevent joint compression and move freely.

6. With even inhales and exhales, continue to keep the shoulders moving away from your ears. You should feel as if your shoulder blades are gliding down your back. Raise your elbows so they are in line with your shoulders. Move your hands away from your face. Try to stay with this posture for 5 breaths, raising your elbows back to shoulder height when they start to drop.
7. After 5 to 10 extended breaths, release your arms and switch so the opposite arm is on top.
8. Repeat steps 3 to 6.
9. Tell your upper body *you're welcome!* and get back to knitting.

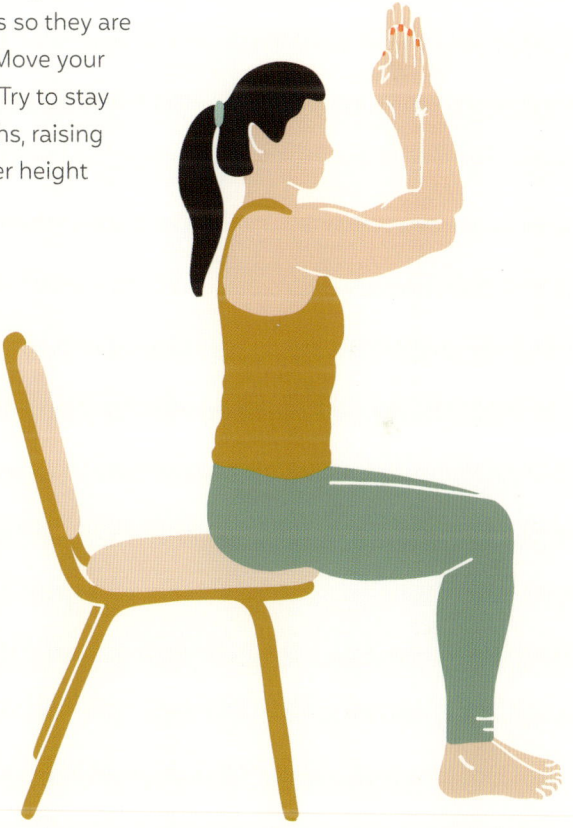

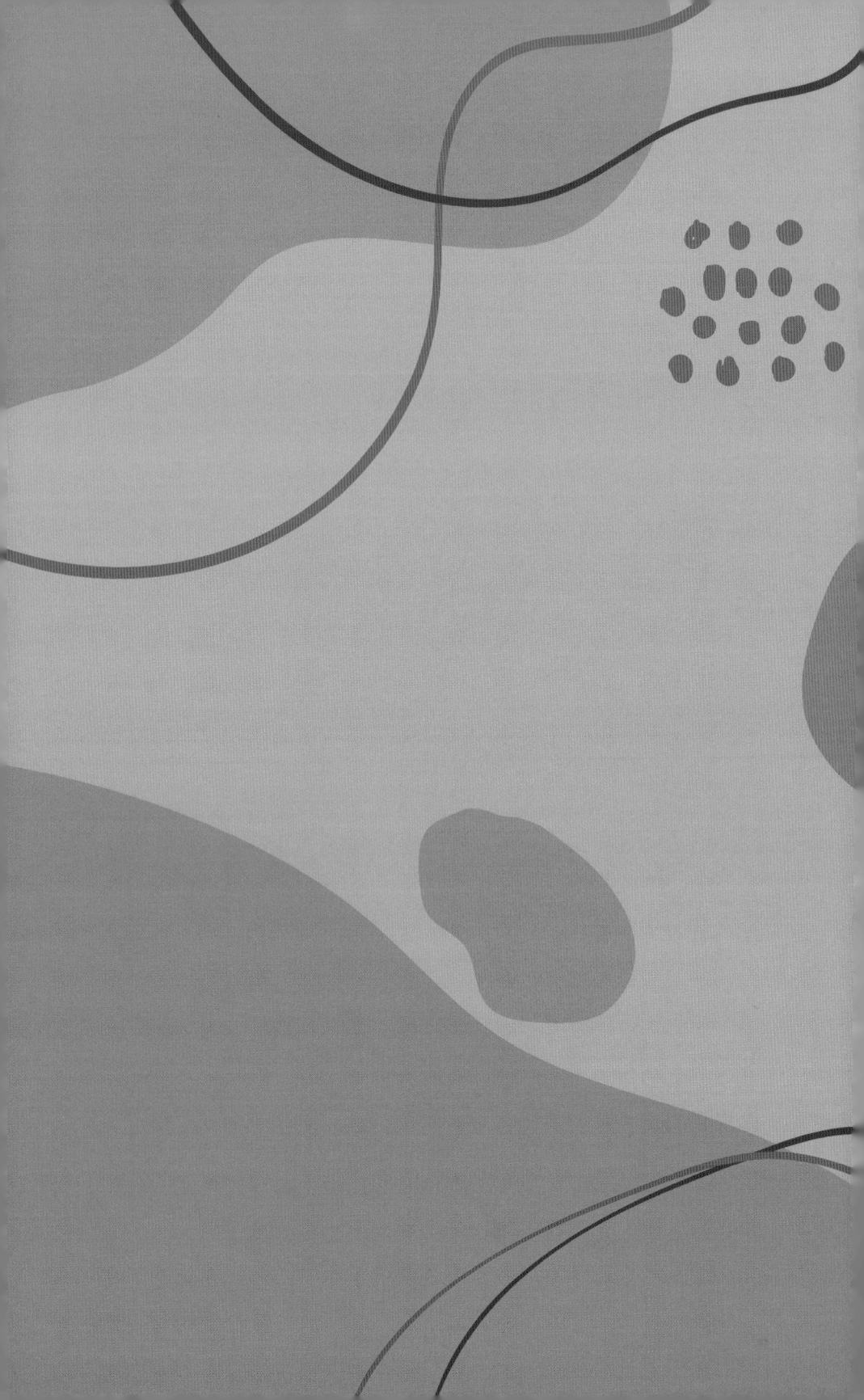

PART THREE

Practice

Here I introduce the philosophy behind practice and its relationship to nonattachment. Practice is repeatedly performing a skill to learn how to do it. Nonattachment is releasing the need to control or fixate on outcomes, people, or physical things. If we integrate practice and nonattachment, we grow with ease, grace, and beauty.

SUTRA 1.14

Sa tu dirgha kala nairantarya satka-rasevito drdhabhumih.
Practice comes firmly grounded when well attended to for a long time, without break and in all earnestness.

DAILY REPETITION

In a nutshell, practice, practice again, and, oh, practice some more! Yoga, meditation, and knitting all take time, patience, and earnestness to learn. It really is that *simple*. But this doesn't necessarily mean it's *easy*. It requires foresight and planning. It requires flexibility. And it requires tradeoffs and sacrifice.

If we can find just five minutes *each and every day*—or as close to that as we can manage—then we will start noticing shifts in our lives. Confidence increases. Our mood improves. Tension in our knitting evens out. Problems that would have thrown us off balance in the past somehow seem more manageable.

But if we miss a day, or two, or three, the benefits slowly start to dissolve, usually before we notice. We later realize we need to get back to it. Anything we earn, we earn through daily repetition. Anything we lose, we lose through lack of it.

We can spend hours reading and philosophizing, but yoga happens when we put in the work. In the same way, we can spend hours reading knitting magazines and browsing thousands of patterns on Ravelry, but ultimately, we learn to knit by knitting. This is a big part of why I think of this book as something we do and not something we merely read.

This sutra teaches us to practice habitually, fervently, and continually. There is no specific amount of time. When we do this, we will notice shifts in our minds and bodies.

CRAVINGS

With daily repetition yoga, meditation, and knitting become non-negotiable habits that serve us well, like brushing our teeth morning and night. We even start to crave these activities. Fortunately, unlike potentially unhealthy cravings—like for sweets, drugs, or alcohol, which can have diminishing returns over time and create dependencies that wreak havoc on our minds, bodies, and relationships—these cravings are good for us.

Yoga, meditation, and knitting are like breathing air. They never run out, and we never need to come down from the high they give us.

YOGA, MEDITATION, AND KNITTING ARE LIKE BREATHING AIR. THEY NEVER RUN OUT, AND WE NEVER NEED TO COME DOWN FROM THE HIGH THEY GIVE US.

IF WE CAN FIND JUST FIVE MINUTES TO PRACTICE EVERY DAY, THEN WE WILL START NOTICING SHIFTS IN OUR LIVES.

BEGIN WHERE WE ARE

I vividly recall the first time I saw a woman in a yoga class transition from a wide-legged-forward-fold into a tripod headstand. I was so excited I immediately tried to copy her. Although I was a beginner, I expected to be able to make this transition from standing on my feet to standing on my head smoothly, which of course didn't happen. Once I got over my frustration, I dedicated myself to practicing the components of that transition. First, build stability and flexibility. Then practice with props and support from a teacher. That is when I began to understand the concept of *begin where you are*. I learned to take things step by step.

We begin where we are because if we try to begin anywhere else, we encounter resistance, which can lead to frustration and discourage our growth. Now, some of us are just go-getters. We want to learn a headstand now—or we want our first sweater to be a steeked colorwork cardigan, and we will accept nothing less. If that rings true, then by all means go forth and conquer. The principle of beginning where we are isn't meant to hold us back. It's intended as a reminder to be honest and kind with ourselves about where we are and also to be realistic about the steps we need to take to grow. We can't wish ourselves into a handstand, but we can dedicate ourselves to learning the skills required, one step at a time. Sometimes, in our eagerness to reach a goal, we try to skip a few steps, which can actually end up slowing us down. When we find ourselves in that situation, we summon the courage to start over and proceed more methodically, which will usually serve us better in the long run.

> WE BEGIN WHERE WE ARE BECAUSE IF WE TRY TO BEGIN ANYWHERE ELSE, WE ENCOUNTER RESISTANCE.

ONE STITCH AT A TIME

After my single mastectomy, I was eager to get right back into practicing yoga to prove to myself that cancer couldn't change me. Then my expectations collided with reality. No one who experiences cancer is unchanged.

For the first six weeks after surgery, I wasn't allowed to lift my right arm above my shoulder, which obviously inhibited my upper body movement. I was frustrated, but I knew the only constructive way forward was to explore within the space I was given. So I meditated and began doing very simple stretches with a chair. I focused on linking my breath with my movements to find greater ease. When I began to knit, I realized that if I engaged in simple breathing practices at the same time, I became much more comfortable and relaxed.

This experience taught me there's always somewhere to begin—whether we're facing a major physical or mental setback, picking up knitting after a decades-long absence, or dealing with anything else life throws our way—as long as we take it one stitch, or one step, at a time.

> **WHEN FACING A CHALLENGE, WE CAN ALWAYS FIND A PLACE TO BEGIN—AS LONG AS WE REMIND OURSELVES TO TAKE IT ONE STITCH, OR ONE STEP, AT A TIME.**

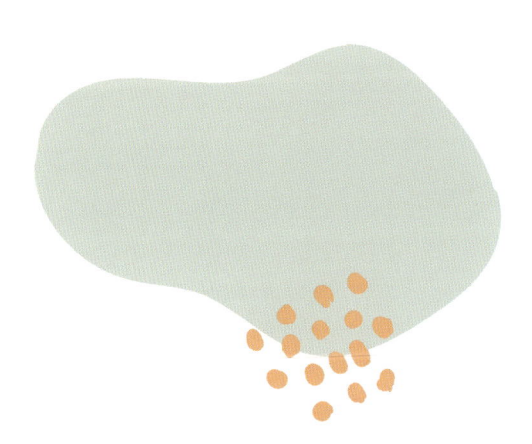

PRACTICE

STICKING TO IT

Even with a daily yoga practice, there are times when focusing the mind or even sitting up straight are challenging. Similarly, even when we knit every day, there are moments when we feel like we're not progressing as quickly as we'd like. Perhaps we're frogging (ripping out stitches) more than we're making them. When these inevitable feelings arise, it's important to treat ourselves kindly. And it's important to stick with our practice.

Progression in yoga and knitting is not always linear. We go back and forth, do a few circles here and there, loop back, and ramble off in one direction, then another. Sometimes we churn out projects one after the other and are able to hold Tree Pose (page 38) indefinitely. At other times, finishing even a single project or holding Tree Pose for just a few seconds feels impossible. Regardless, it's our job to show up daily. If we do that and put in the work, the benefits come. And the benefits we experience touch every aspect of our lives.

No effort is ever wasted when we are working on our craft. Any time we spend resting in Child's Pose, practicing our breathing, knitting a few stitches, or tinking (unknitting) those same stitches, adds up. The amount of time we spend knitting or meditating each day isn't our main focus. The size of a finished object doesn't determine its quality. What matters is how fully we can focus our attention during that experience.

We benefit when we're open to trying new approaches, especially ones that we naturally avoid. A bit of contrary action is necessary to any good daily practice in order to make discoveries and build up our yoga and knitting toolkits. At least some days, think about the thing you want to practice the least, and then go do it!

> IT'S OUR JOB TO SHOW UP DAILY. IF WE DO THAT AND PUT IN THE WORK, THE BENEFITS COME. AND THE BENEFITS WE EXPERIENCE TOUCH EVERY ASPECT OF OUR LIVES.

SEATED TWIST

Seated Twist, *parivrtta sukhasana*, is a posture that all knitters need. Twisting before and after a knitting session will not only clear your mind, it will also release tension and toxins from the body. Twists are all about creating space.

Benefits: Releases tension in the neck, shoulders, and back. **Prop:** Chair

If you have a back, shoulder, or neck injury, avoid this posture.

1. Sit with your bottom on the edge of the chair. Plant your feet on the floor hip distance apart.
2. Reach your arms up overhead as you inhale deeply through your nose. If an injury prevents you from lifting your arms overhead, then leave them down as you turn.
3. Twist to the right as you exhale through your mouth. Place your left hand on your right knee and your right hand onto the chair behind you to deepen the twist. The twist happens in the mid to upper back. Try not to move your hips, knees, or legs. Keep your chin parallel to the floor and your gaze forward. Only turn your neck to look over your right shoulder if you can do so without resistance.
4. Count 3 inhales and exhales in the twist.
5. Reach your arms up overhead as you inhale through your nose and turn back to center.

Repeat steps 3–5, turning to the opposite side, placing your right hand on your left knee and your left hand on the back of the chair.

WHEN WE RELEASE THE NEED TO CONTROL OR FORCE OUR KNITTING, WE OPEN OURSELVES UP TO ENJOYING EACH STITCH FOR ITS OWN SAKE.

IMPERMANENCE

While pregnant with my second child, I had the urge to design and knit a round brioche baby blanket. I already had my hands full and plenty of other projects still on the needles, but the urge was strong, so I went with it. I designed and knit an entire 36" (91 cm) round baby blanket with intricate increases and decreases, and I even bound off to the last stitch. Then I took a good look at it and ripped out the entire thing! The colors weren't right, and there was a mistake halfway through. This was probably the first time I unraveled an entire project without feeling any tinge of guilt, remorse, or failure. I realized that this project was more about the act of preparing for the bundle of joy in my belly than having a finished knit for the baby. It was fun to knit. I enjoyed the process, and I satisfied my urge. I never became committed to the permanence of the finished blanket.

When we release the need to control or force our knitting, we open ourselves up to enjoying each stitch for its own sake. If we show up to our meditation practice with an intention to sit for 10 minutes, but then our dog tries to sit on our lap or our kids run in screaming, we can choose how to react. Perhaps we meditate through the noise, or we calmly pause and revisit later.

When we practice nonattachment, we show respect to everything else in the world that has its own desires, plans, and goals. And we become open to learning from them, especially when they impinge on our own goals.

NONATTACHMENT

Our ability to quiet our minds comes when we are no longer clinging to our desires or cravings for material goods. Despite what our consumer culture tells us every day, a life propelled by a need for material objects can never be a fulfilling one. Advertisers regularly try to convince us that their products—a new car, the latest shade of lipstick, or a particular credit card—will bring us happiness. But what they leave out is that none of the pleasure these items bring us will endure. When our mental, emotional, and physical energy is directed toward obtaining something we believe we want or need in order to be happy, our thoughts are clouded by those desires, and we miss out on what we have now.

Nonattachment still can happen while enjoying material things in life. We do not need to give up all of our worldly possessions and go live in a cave.

I enjoy my yarn, knits, delicious cheeses, and yummy baked goods, and I am eyeing a new set of interchangeable needles. But I do not let these items determine my emotional well-being.

When practicing nonattachment, we strive not to direct all our mental energy to acquiring new things or clinging to those we have. We certainly can be disappointed when we lose a cherished object or don't get something we want—especially certain skeins of yarn! But it never pushes us off balance. It doesn't affect who we are or how we find meaning. We can practice yoga and remember that we are calm, strong warriors of kindness who find meaning in our own self-growth and the positive energy we bring to our relationships. And we can do all this without renouncing our homes and everything in them.

> DESPITE WHAT OUR CONSUMER CULTURE TELLS US EVERY DAY, A LIFE PROPELLED BY A NEED FOR MATERIAL OBJECTS CAN NEVER BE A FULFILLING ONE.

STASH STATUS

Now we come to a rather contentious issue in the knitting community. How does this idea of nonattachment apply to our yarn stashes? It's simple: We don't need to hoard yarn! But we also don't need to give all our yarn away. Like most things in life, the answer is somewhere between the extremes. We want to establish a kind of freedom from clinging to our yarn and related notions in unhealthy ways. At the same time, we can enjoy what we have.

> WE HAVE ACHIEVED SABLE STATUS WHEN WE HAVE ACCUMULATED MORE YARN THAN WE COULD EVER POSSIBLY KNIT IN THE REMAINING TIME WE HAVE ON EARTH.

So let's start small. First, we should ask ourselves if we have attained SABLE status. SABLE means *Stash Acquired Beyond Life Expectancy*. We have achieved SABLE status when we have accumulated more yarn than we could ever possibly knit in the remaining time we have on Earth. If you've achieved SABLE status, then your next step is simple. Take a moment to jump for joy, roll around in your yarn, and love it! Then donate a healthy portion of it to your knitter friends or a local guild, library, or school. Don't think too hard about it. If the yarn can be useful to someone else, hand it over with no strings attached.

Of course, even if we haven't reached SABLE status, many of us acquire more yarn than we need. It's good to get into the habit of assessing what we have compared to what we need

SUTRA 1.15

Drstanusravika visaya vitrsnasya vasikara samjna vairagyam.

The consciousness of self-mastery in one who is free from craving for objects seen or heard about is nonattachment.

on a regular basis. Once we do this assessment, we might decide to begin a donation pile. For years I lived in a small city apartment, and my stash was tucked into nooks and crannies due to lack of space. This made it hard for me to take stock of it and figure out what to use for a new project, what to give away to a friend, and what I wanted to hold onto because I had big dreams for it.

Now I live in a roomy home in the country where I have set up my very own wall of yarn in my bedroom. I regularly rearrange it, giving my current favorite skeins and finished objects prime placement, and pulling out and giving away yarn I think might be better used by another knitter. As long as I do this every so often, I don't feel guilty about buying new skeins that call to me or about the size of my stash overall. I'm a yarn lover, and I'm not afraid to admit it!

GIVING BACK

When considering your stash, it's also important to think about giving back. When I was being treated for breast cancer, I found solace in knitting hats for my fellow patients at Mass General Hospital. I followed one pattern in a few different sizes and placed the hats on the donation table in the chemotherapy waiting area. Giving to others who, like me, didn't have a lick of hair on their heads felt really good.

There are so many charities and hospitals that will accept handknits. And there are so many people out there who will appreciate the love we stitch into them. Just keep in mind that it's usually best to knit with machine-washable yarn that can handle wear and tear, or to clearly label the items with care instructions. When in doubt, check with the organization to which you would like to donate.

RESETS

Once our yoga, meditation, or knitting feels like a natural extension of daily life, and we're used to practicing at home, it becomes second nature to fit in time here and there to enjoy what we love. The more time we dedicate, the more we'll be able to recreate this feeling of joy no matter where we are or how little time we have.

RESETTING WITH MUDRAS

On days when I feel mentally foggy, when I'm having trouble concentrating, I will typically take some deep breaths as a way to reset my body and mind. If that isn't enough, I turn to these mudras. I think of these breaks as the mental equivalent of turning my computer off and on again to get rid of the kinks. Remember: We can reset our days and start fresh whenever and as often as we choose.

FIVE FACES GESTURE, *panchamukha mudra*

Benefits: Enhances memory retention and improves concentration.
Props: Chair, timer

If you have a hand or wrist injury, avoid this posture.

1. Sitting in a chair, set your timer for 5 minutes.
2. Bring your hands together in front of your belly so all 5 fingertips touch each other, leaving a space between your palms, as though you have an imaginary ball of yarn between them.
3. Let the breath push your abdomen in and out. Notice the thoughts that arise. Relax the jaw. Coax the shoulders away from the ears.
4. Keep breathing with hands in this position until the timer goes off.

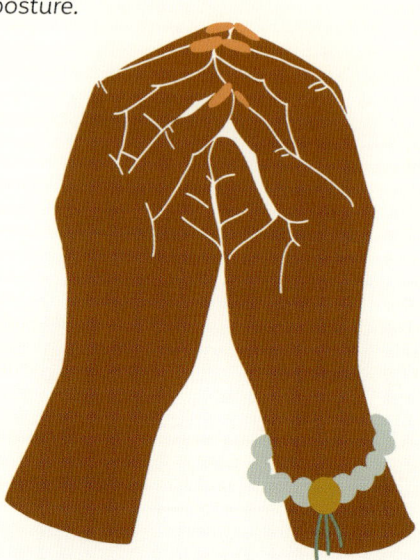

Small breaks for meditation or yoga can give the same sense of accomplishment and grounding as a 90-minute session. Only a few stitches or rows, or just a few minutes in Child's Pose (page 42), can help us achieve an inner equilibrium and refresh us for whatever challenges lie ahead.

SEAL OF WISDOM, *jnana mudra*

Benefits: Brings us back to our center and helps us find inner wisdom.
Props: Chair or folded blanket, timer

If you have a hand or wrist injury, avoid this posture.

1. Sit in a chair or cross-legged on a folded blanket on the floor. Set a timer for 5 minutes.
2. Place the backs of your hands on your upper thighs, with palms facing up.
3. Join the tips of your thumb and index finger on each hand. Leave your remaining fingers extended and relaxed. Inhale and exhale through your nose. Relax your shoulders away from your ears.
4. Focus on steady inhales and exhales. As new thoughts arise, bring the awareness back to the connection of the thumb and index finger.
5. When the timer goes off, shake out your hands and slowly transition back to your day.

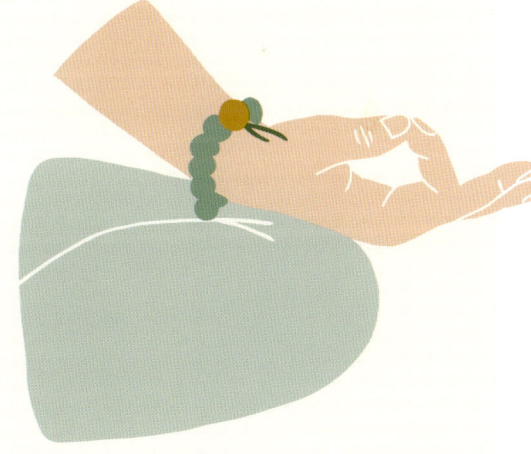

WORK IN PROGRESS

In the knitting community, we sometimes call a project we haven't finished yet a *WIP*, or a *Work in Progress*. I like to think of our bodies and minds as perpetual WIPs. Taking this perspective opens up new freedoms. We learn to accept mistakes and recognize that they are opportunities for discovery. We learn to be playful in everything we do; we lose the rush to completion that is so ingrained in our society.

When we take a yoga class, a teacher leads us through a sequence of poses, typically for 60 or 90 minutes. We follow along as best we can. But yoga doesn't stop when we walk out the studio door. Our bodies keep moving. Intentionally or unintentionally, we take on postures that either trap tension or release it. Each moment our bodies are in a posture that either serves us or harms us, whether we are paying attention or not. We can always find something to explore in our bodies and minds, even if it's just noticing what our current posture is and whether it's serving us or not. In this very practical sense, our work as yogis is never done.

As we grow as yogis, we begin to appreciate how naïve it is to think this journey could ever reach a destination. We see how deep and broad yoga is, how its teachings stretch far beyond the boundaries of a single human lifetime.

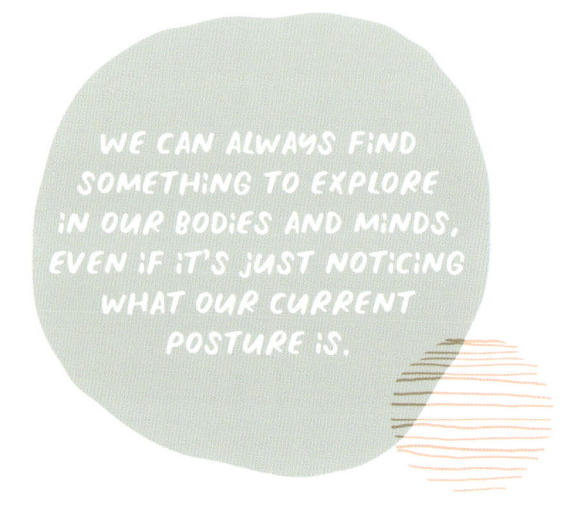

> WE CAN ALWAYS FIND SOMETHING TO EXPLORE IN OUR BODIES AND MINDS, EVEN IF IT'S JUST NOTICING WHAT OUR CURRENT POSTURE IS.

KNITTING AND YOGA STYLES

As modern knitters, we know we have seemingly endless choices in yarns, notions, and projects. Maybe we like breezing through a project with bulky yarn and big needles on a rocking chair on our porch. Maybe we like knitting with double-pointed needles in trains, airplanes, and waiting rooms. Personally, I like to have a bunch of projects going at once, each serving a different mood or desire.

Yoga is no different from knitting. There are myriad approaches. It's up to each of us to find the ones that fulfill us, remembering that we may need something different on different days or during different periods of our lives. Some days my body is craving a vigorous *Ashtanga* practice. This is a highly energetic practice for when I need to get the wiggles out. Other days I need a *Bhakti* practice. This is a devotional prayer and chanting practice to help foster unconditional love and reset my attitude toward life. Still other days I need *Kundalini*, a yoga style with more spiritual leanings, or *Iyengar*, a practice that focuses on precision, alignment, and honing attention to detail.

This life is all one big practice during which we can always continue learning and growing. If we can hold onto our beginner's mind and practice daily, new styles of knitting and yoga will call out to us. We just have to tune in and have the courage to explore. If it feels right, it is right. And if the path ends up leading us somewhere we didn't expect—somewhere that doesn't fit with our preconceptions—let's ask what the universe was trying to tell us rather than regret the decisions we've made.

> WE BENEFIT WHEN WE'RE OPEN TO TRYING NEW APPROACHES, ESPECIALLY ONES THAT WE NATURALLY AVOID.

WHAT'S YOUR KNITTING AND YOGA STYLE?

Our Western culture too often displays a caricature of yoga where beautiful people in perfect postures glisten through an intense *Vinyasa* class. I love breaking a sweat as much as the next yogi, but yoga is so much more than that. It can support your life no matter your age or physical condition. To realize these benefits, it helps to let go of stereotypes and explore different forms of yoga to figure out what resonates for us.

Type of Knitting	Relationship of Type of Knitting to Yoga Styles
Scarves	Scarves and *Hatha* yoga bring us back to basics without complication. Just as we might make a garter-stitch or ribbed scarf to ground ourselves, we can return to the basic poses of *Hatha* for the same effect.
Shawls	Shawls and *Restorative* yoga are slower-paced and encourage us to breathe, take our time, and explore without pressure or expectation. Shawls are also great to wear during a *Restorative* practice as we warm and rest the body.
Projects Worked in the Round	Projects worked in the round have a rhythm and flow to them as each stitch builds on the prior stitch to create a wonderful garment. In *Vinyasa* a similar build-up occurs through rhythm and flow.
Cables	Cables and *Yin* yoga both require patience and perseverance in a slow, repetitive process.

To entice you, I have created a fun, slightly tongue-in-cheek chart that highlights the links between different yoga and knitting styles. This is by no means an exhaustive list. It's intended only to encourage and guide you toward exploring new ways to engage your body and mind.

Yoga Style	Yoga Description
Hatha	*Hatha* yoga is the foundation of the physical poses we know in America today. *Ha* means *sun* and *tha* means *moon*. Yoga means to *yoke* or *unite*. The sun refers to the active masculine, and the moon refers to the receptive feminine aspects in all of us. Thus, *Hatha* yoga is the journey toward the unification and balance of the masculine and feminine. Most *Hatha* classes involve a basic introduction to yoga.
Restorative	*Restorative* yoga focuses on resting in a limited number of poses for a long time with the support of props like blocks, blankets, or bolsters, so our bodies can relax fully.
Vinyasa	*Vinyasa* is a flow style of yoga where postures are linked by breath. The postures build on one another step by step as the breath moves the body.
Yin	*Yin* is a very slow-paced yoga where we hold postures for extended periods of time to find deeper relaxation and ease.

(continued on next page)

(continued from previous page)

Type of Knitting	Relationship of Type of Knitting to Yoga Styles
Stranded Knitting	Stranded, or fair isle knitting, and *Ashtanga* yoga both emphasize a particular sequencing that requires a single-pointed focus and dedication.
Lightweight Non-Animal Fiber Yarns	Knitters who enjoy working with cotton, linen, or silk to create lightweight garments may find a similar challenge in *Bikram* yoga or hot yoga. Your body will expand just like your cotton stitches in the extreme heat.
Socks or Leg Warmers	Knitting socks or leg warmers requires repetition, an important aspect of the *Kundalini* system for activating internal power.
Prayer Shawls	Practicing *Bhakti* yoga and knitting prayer shawls are both devotional practices of love.
Projects Knit for Donation	Knitting for charity and *Karma* yoga both focus on service to others.

Yoga Style	Yoga Description
Ashtanga	In this mentally and physically demanding practice, we do the exact same poses in the exact same order every time.
Bikram/Hot	In *Bikram* yoga, we always do the same 26 poses in the same order in a heated room. Hot yoga is heated yoga but without *Bikram's* sequence of 26 poses. Many hot yoga classes are *Vinyasa* style. The heat in both of these styles is used to clear out toxins and intensify the experience.
Kundalini	*Kundalini* is the spiritual energy located at the base of your spine. *Kundalini* yoga includes repetitive movements, breathing exercises, chants, and songs to activate the *Kundalini* energy within.
Bhakti	*Bhakti* yoga is the devotional practice of universal love. The Western manifestation of *Bhakti* yoga and devotion focuses on chanting while filling your heart with love and beauty.
Karma	*Karma* yoga is the yoga of action, taking the yoga philosophy off the mat and living it through service to others.

MENTAL FLEXIBILITY

Physical flexibility comes and goes with our daily repetition, or lack thereof. But mental flexibility, which can relieve emotional suffering, has a stronger long-term memory.

Mental flexibility helps us place ourselves in counterfactuals, meaning we can put ourselves in someone else's shoes, imagine what it would be like if a situation were different, or try out ideas that aren't typical for us. Being open to the possibility of change helps us adjust to new situations and perspectives with ease and comfort.

We can build up mental flexibility in our knitting and yoga and translate this adaptability to every aspect of our lives. Imagine arriving at a yoga class and realizing someone has taken your favorite spot in the back right corner. Are you annoyed, or do you see this as a way to find a new "home" and gain a new perspective? Maybe you start knitting a colorwork hat. As you knit, you find the cast-on is too tight. Do you try to convince yourself that the cast-on will loosen when blocked, even though experience tells you it probably won't budge? Or do you have the courage and flexibility to start over? How long it takes us to realize we need to change course, and how smoothly we make the change, are signs of our mental flexibility—or lack thereof.

Mental flexibility is not one of my natural strengths, so I have to work on it continuously. For example, a couple of years ago I bought a one-of-a-kind skein of bulky variegated handspun yarn with the intention of making a vest for my daughter. It turned out I was asking the universe to teach me a lesson. I cast on and started the vest only to realize I didn't have enough yarn. I was dead-set on this being a one-skein project, so I knew I had to rip it out and start something new.

> HOW LONG IT TAKES US TO REALIZE WE NEED TO CHANGE COURSE, AND HOW SMOOTHLY WE MAKE THE CHANGE, ARE SIGNS OF OUR MENTAL FLEXIBILITY—OR LACK THEREOF.

YOGA OF YARN

To my credit, I started over right away—this time with the idea of making a poncho. About five inches in, I realized the fabric was too stiff for a poncho and, again, that I didn't have enough yarn. I dropped the needles, cussed under my breath, and walked away.

A few days later, I let my eyes peek at the project again, and it just popped into my head that this yarn would make a nice bolster for my yoga practice. I let go of the idea that I had to knit something for my daughter, and I unraveled the fabric to start anew. It knit up very nicely and quickly once I was working on the right project. But it had taken me days to let go of my own expectations for the skein. During that period, I needlessly suffered through my own mind's lack of flexibility. Now I try to use that experience and many others like it as assets to help me stay mentally flexible in all kinds of situations.

> WE CAN BUILD UP MENTAL FLEXIBILITY IN OUR KNITTING AND YOGA AND TRANSLATE THIS ADAPTABILITY TO EVERY ASPECT OF OUR LIVES.

FLEXIBLE BOLSTER

I designed this bolster with yarn I originally bought to make a vest for my daughter. I take it with me to knitting group meetups and use it as a support for my back. It's also wonderful for my home yoga practice when I do Supported Fish Pose on the floor.

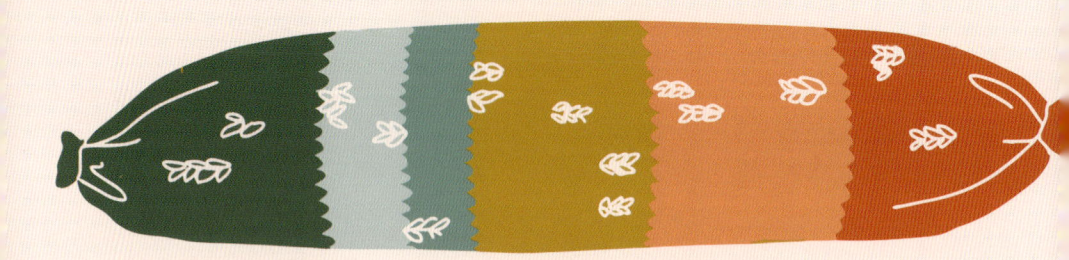

Size & Dimensions
23" (58 cm) long by 14" (36 cm) circumference

Materials
92 yards (84 meters) bulky-weight variegated yarn

Scrap yarn for provisional cast-on, stitch marker, pillow stuffing

Size US 11 (8 mm) 16" (40 cm) circular needle, or size needed to obtain gauge

Gauge
8 stitches and 14 rounds = 4" (10 cm) in Stockinette stitch (knit every round), after blocking

Always use a needle size that will result in the correct gauge after blocking.

Bolster
Cast on 27 stitches using scrap yarn and provisional cast-on. Join in the round, being careful not to twist stitches. Place a marker at the beginning of the round.

Work in Stockinette stitch (knit every round) until piece measures 23" (58 cm) from the cast-on edge. Cut the yarn, leaving an 8" (20 cm) tail.

With a tapestry needle, thread the tail through the stitches and pull tight to close the end.

Fill with pillow stuffing to desired firmness.

Unravel the provisional cast-on. With a tapestry needle and a strand of yarn 10" (25.5 cm) long, thread the yarn through the live stitches and pull tight to close the end; tie the ends together in a double knot to secure them.

Weave in the ends.

YOGA OF YARN

SUPPORTED FISH POSE

Supported Fish Pose, *matsyasana*, is a wonderful place to take stock of your body. I find it especially helpful to open my chest, relax my shoulders, and ease my breath after a long knitting session.

Benefits: Opens the chest, relieves tension in the neck and shoulders, and improves posture. **Props:** Bolster

If you have a back injury, avoid this posture.

1. Place the bolster on the floor. Sit in front of the bolster with your knees bent and feet flat on the floor. The bolster will be horizontal to your body.

2. Take your hands behind you on the floor and lower yourself back down until the tips of your shoulder blades are touching the bolster. Lie all the way back so your chest feels lifted and supported and the back of your head rests on the floor. Breathe deeply in this position for at least 20 breaths, checking in with each part of your body, starting with your toes and progressing to your ankles, shins, calves, knees, quads, hamstrings, hips, sacrum, lower back, belly, chest, shoulders, upper arms, forearms, wrists, fingers, neck, and head. Focus your attention on each of these parts as you inhale and exhale. Ask them how they are doing, maybe wiggle them gently, and see if they have anything to tell you.

3. Stay here or straighten your legs.

4. When you are ready to transition out of the posture, roll with care to one side and press your hands gently into the floor to rise. Make your way to standing and go about your day.

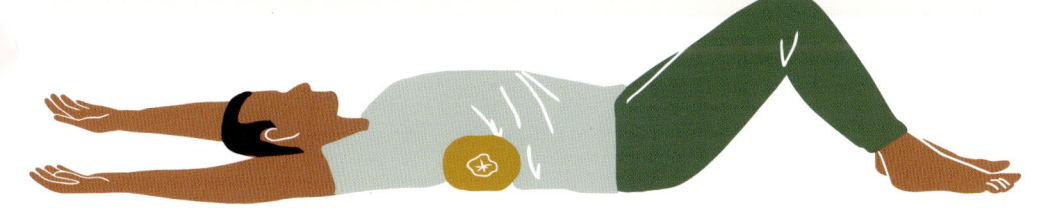

ANYTIME, ANYWHERE

One of the many wonderful qualities that knitting and yoga share is that they can be practiced anytime, anywhere. To do yoga, we only need ourselves. To knit, we only need to add some needles and yarn. This means we can always stay on track with a project and keep our bodies and minds flexible no matter where we are in the world.

To be ready when the moment strikes, I suggest you make note of a few of your favorite movements and meditations you feel comfortable doing in public. I also suggest you always carry a knitting project with you. You never know when you'll be stuck somewhere and eager to make good use of the time.

Following these suggestions is not too difficult most days. It's not all that challenging to find space in a bag for a small knitting project. But what about longer work trips or family vacations? Here are seven tips to help keep your knitting and yoga practices alive—so you don't risk losing the benefits of your daily practice—when your daily routine is disrupted.

> MAKE NOTE OF A FEW OF YOUR FAVORITE MOVEMENTS AND MEDITATIONS YOU FEEL COMFORTABLE DOING IN PUBLIC, SO YOU'RE READY WHEN THE MOMENT STRIKES.

1. UNDERWEAR IS OVERRATED.

I've taken too many trips where I packed not one but three knitting projects and not a single piece of underwear. You might think I would regret this decision; instead, I stand by my belief that underwear is overrated. There really is no need to pack it. I can easily run to a shop and buy cheap undies pretty much anywhere in the world. Yarn, however, is not always so easy to find.

2. PACK AT LEAST ONE SMALL PROJECT IN YOUR CARRY-ON.

If you're traveling by plane, pack a simple one-skein project in your carry-on. You can pull it out during the many times you will be asked to wait patiently—in a line, in a waiting area, on the plane. One exception: If you're taking a really long flight and/or are lucky enough to be flying in business or first class where you can stretch out, you may feel comfortable working on something larger or more complex. I once tried to work on a brioche project in coach in a middle seat, and it ended up being so stressful that I've never wanted to try it again.

3. YOU GOTTA HAVE OPTIONS.

So you're packing for a relaxing vacation and you want to make sure you have options. You already have your small project for your carry-on, but what about your suitcase? I try to pack one project for a two- to four-day trip, two projects for a week-long trip, and two or three projects for a two-week trip, plus a set of interchangeable needles. If I've scouted out yarn shops in the area I'm visiting, then I may pack fewer projects because I know I'm likely to pick up something new!

4. PLAN FOR THE SECURITY CHECKPOINT.

Years ago my mom and I flew to Costa Rica together. I tucked my knitting and notions bag into my carry-on, but I forgot to transfer a special pair of gold crane scissors to my suitcase before checking in. The TSA officer found them as I was going through security and told me to throw them away. While I was pleading with him to let me keep them, an extremely nice man passing the other way offered to take the scissors and mail them back to me. And he actually did! I still feel grateful the universe arranged for that man to pass by at that very moment.

Since that Costa Rica trip, every time I travel I bring a pre-addressed manila envelope with two or three forever stamps on it in case I need to mail myself anything. Luckily, I haven't needed it, but it comforts me to know that some silly mishap won't result in my nice needles meeting the bottom of an airport trash bin. The pre-stamped envelope only works while in one's home-country airports, of course.

In addition, I travel with cheap TSA-approved scissors, and I try to stick with plastic or wooden needles in my carry-on since they seem to raise fewer eyebrows than metal ones. Technically, knitting needles are TSA-approved, but every now and then you come across an agent who doesn't realize this and will confiscate them no matter how confidently you attempt to explain the rule.

5. PROTECT YOUR VALUABLES.

To protect all of my yarn and knitwear, I pack them in resealable plastic bags or even small, clean garbage bags. Before sealing, I sit on them to remove air and save space. I also pack extra bags in case I buy some yarn during my travels. While I was living in Los Angeles, I took a trip to Rosehaven Alpacas in the Catskills in New York and fell in love with their popcorn yarn. It's a good thing I put it in a protective bag because a shampoo bottle exploded on the way home, and it wasn't pretty!

6. PACK A BALL OR TWO.

When I travel to teach, I like to bring my own lightweight yoga mat, but when I'm vacationing I leave my mat at home. Instead, I use what is available to me at the hotel where I'm staying. Usually, there is a chair and a spare towel that can act as a yoga mat, or I just practice right on the floor. One yoga prop I like to pack is a tennis or lacrosse ball. Hours of sitting in a car or on a plane build tension all over, and having a ball handy gives me a chance to check in with myself and work out any kinks.

7. MARK YOUR CALENDAR.

A little planning and some gentle reminders on your calendar will keep you on track with your daily practices. When I travel, I schedule five-minute yoga and meditation sessions for the morning and evening. If my trip isn't jam-packed with other events, I adjust as I go and add in more time.

> TO PROTECT ALL OF MY YARN AND KNITWEAR, I PACK THEM IN RESEALABLE PLASTIC BAGS OR EVEN SMALL, CLEAN GARBAGE BAGS.

TRANSITIONS

Knitting is a practice of transitions. We switch from purl to knit, ribbing to stockinette stitch, and brioche to garter. When we are learning these transitions, we slow down and focus on what we're doing. But after a little while, the new movements feel as natural as breathing. The same happens in yoga. When we learn Sun Salutations (page 156), shifting from one posture to the next can feel clunky. But we begin slowly. We time the movements with our breathing. Our body learns the rhythm, and we follow it.

Smooth transitions mean our daily repetition is paying off. We are growing. The more we do this in our knitting and yoga, the more we start to notice that we can smoothly transition in other parts of our lives as well. Life is sure to throw us challenges, but we are ready for them. We can transition smoothly out of one set of circumstances and into another.

When I was diagnosed with breast cancer, my ability to transition was put to the test. At first I cried a lot, which makes sense since crying is a natural physiological response to increased stress hormones. Then I turned to yoga, meditation, and journaling to help me slow down and move into a new reality that included surgery and chemotherapy. Meditation helped me process my emotions without judgment. Yoga helped my body release tension and rebuild strength and flexibility. Knitting and journaling helped me pass the time productively and quiet my mind.

> **WHEN WE ARE LEARNING THESE TRANSITIONS, WE SLOW DOWN AND FOCUS ON WHAT WE'RE DOING. BUT AFTER A LITTLE WHILE, THE NEW MOVEMENTS FEEL AS NATURAL AS BREATHING.**

Whether we are moving from knit to purl or from healthy to sick, it helps to acknowledge these common stages.

1. We need to admit to ourselves that a transition is happening. No matter how obvious it might be, we need to take a moment to explicitly acknowledge it.

2. We need to ask ourselves what previously held expectations are now being shattered. The sooner we remind ourselves that life offers no guarantee of fulfilling our expectations, the less resistant we will be to the transition.

3. We need to exercise some mental flexibility and ask ourselves how we could benefit if we looked at this transition another way. If the transition is very hard, this might be tough to do, but we need to try. To help, we might recall anxiety we felt during past transitions and ask ourselves if that anxiety turned out to be necessary or helpful. Or we might reach out to friends and family. By talking about our thoughts and feelings, we can neutralize the negative impact they have on us.

And then we can let time do the rest. We will grow with this transition, no matter how impossible it may seem in the moment. Remember this helpful mantra: *Today is the tomorrow we were afraid of yesterday.*

> **WE NEED TO ADMIT TO OURSELVES THAT A TRANSITION IS HAPPENING. NO MATTER HOW OBVIOUS IT MIGHT BE, WE NEED TO TAKE A MOMENT TO EXPLICITLY ACKNOWLEDGE IT.**

FINDING BALANCE

In each yoga posture we strive to achieve a unification of opposites, a balance between strength, which requires a certain degree of rigidity, and comfort, which calls for suppleness.

Whether we're holding a yoga pose, knitting, or even simply thinking, ideally we are always seeking to find the balance between strength and flexibility.

In a standing posture, we find balance between our feet pressed into the ground and our bodies reaching to the sky. We try not to go too far in one direction or the other, but by testing our limits in each direction, we achieve balance.

We repeat poses for an equal amount of time on the left and right to see how the same body parts on different sides respond. We use the left side of our bodies to evaluate the right side, and vice versa. We do this to restore balance along our three body axes: left and right, front and back, top and bottom.

We do the same with our minds. Thoughts pull our attention into fears about the future and regrets about the past. We can find balance by quieting our minds and bringing our thoughts back to the present moment. We may watch our thoughts to see if our left brain or right brain is dominating.

SUTRA 2.46
Sthira sukhamasanam.

A yoga pose is a steady and comfortable posture.

Are we thinking logically and analytically (left brain)? Or are we thinking creatively and intuitively (right brain)? Are we exhibiting one tendency much more than the other? Can we bring our minds back to balance between their creative and logical functions?

Finding balance between strength and flexibility reminds me of knitting lace. We want our lace to be strong but supple. We create symmetry when we mirror our various increases and decreases. We find balance between the stitches and the empty spaces that form the design. We strive to translate the balance between strength and flexibility in our bodies and our stitches.

> WHETHER WE'RE HOLDING A YOGA POSE, KNITTING, OR EVEN SIMPLY THINKING, IDEALLY WE ARE ALWAYS SEEKING TO FIND THE BALANCE BETWEEN STRENGTH AND FLEXIBILITY.

NOTICING ONE THING

How we do one thing is how we do everything. The first time I heard this adage I immediately thought of an obsessive tendency of mine—when I put my yoga mat on the floor, I adjust it so it's perfectly straight and parallel to the orientation of the room. Once I noticed this habit, I saw other instances when I fixed niggling, perhaps unimportant, inconsistencies and asymmetries. I began to see how this compulsive tendency was distracting me from being in the moment or from going with the flow.

If we can remain in tune with our needs and look out for the common patterns in the little things we do, then we can use those clues to start investigating bigger issues more concretely and with better direction. Eventually, we will learn to ease up and offer more compassion to ourselves and others. Perhaps paradoxically, the more compassion we grant ourselves, the more we are able to notice our negative tendencies, because we are no longer judging them as harshly or holding onto them so intensely.

We can gain insight into our attitudes in the moment by noticing how we hold yoga positions. In all my postures, I generally rely more on strength than flexibility. In my life, I exhibit the same tendency. I hold onto things. I control. I stand my ground. I'm stubborn. This is why I continually work on introducing suppleness into my yoga practice and into my life overall. Like everyone, I am a work in progress, and each day I meet myself where I am. Looking at how I do one thing gives me insight into how I do everything. And that keeps me open to growth in every aspect of my life.

> IF WE CAN REMAIN IN TUNE WITH OUR NEEDS AND LOOK OUT FOR THE COMMON PATTERNS IN THE LITTLE THINGS WE DO, THEN WE CAN USE THOSE CLUES TO START INVESTIGATING BIGGER ISSUES.

HOLDING YOUR NEEDLES

This simple exercise brings awareness to how we hold knitting needles and how that affects the knitting experience. When I knit for an extended period of time without doing this exercise, I tend to build up tension in my hands or neck. When I remember to incorporate this exercise into my knitting routine, it helps me relax.

Benefits: Provides a concrete way to check balance between strength and flexibility at any given moment. **Props:** Chair, yarn, needles

1. Sit down and start knitting. Let your mind wander. After a few minutes, pay attention to how you're holding your needles. Ask and answer these questions to increase awareness of your posture. Don't judge your answers. Just notice and adjust.

   - *Am I gripping the needles more tightly than necessary?*
   - *Am I holding my arms high or low? Where are my elbows?*
   - *Am I pressing the end of the needle into my thigh to steady it?*
   - *Am I leaning more toward strength and rigidity or comfort and flexibility?*
   - *What can I do right now to adjust my balance?*

2. Make your adjustments. Knit for a few more minutes while you let your mind wander. Now go through these steps again.

If possible, repeat this process at least 2 to 4 times during a 20- to 45-minute knitting session. Notice if your hands and arms revert to their initial positioning or not and, if so, how quickly.

TAKING CARE

As knitters, we repeat the same stitches and thus move our bodies in the same ways over and over. In that way, we are like high-performance athletes, so we need to take care of ourselves just like an athlete would.

An important part of our high-performance training is to think beyond the health of our hands and remember that everything is connected in our minds and bodies. This means the repetitive motions of knitting affect not only remote body parts, but also our thoughts.

HAND AND WRIST PREP

Try this sequence of 5 hand and wrist exercises, then pick 2 or 3 to do each and every time you prepare to knit. You can do these sitting or standing.

PALM RUB

Benefits: Warms up the hand muscles. **Props:** None

If you have a wrist or hand injury, avoid this practice.

1. Place your palms together in front of your chest.
2. Rub your palms together in a rapid motion as you slowly count to 10. Feel the warmth building between your palms.

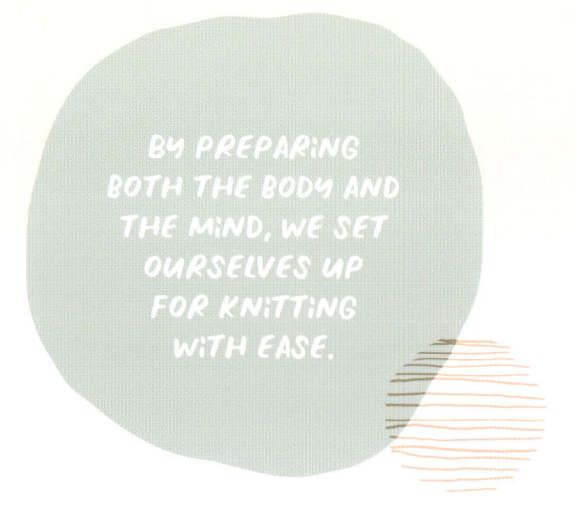

> BY PREPARING BOTH THE BODY AND THE MIND, WE SET OURSELVES UP FOR KNITTING WITH EASE.

For years, I took the health of my hands, wrists, neck, and shoulders for granted. That changed during chemotherapy. The treatment I received continues to affect the nerves in all of my extremities to this day. Yoga has given me a path to maintain my body so I can knit without unbearable numbness or pain. But if I don't put in the work each day, I don't see the benefits. And I pay the price—sometimes not right away, but eventually I always do.

Check out the following movements, choose the ones you think you can benefit from, and try to practice them regularly.

FINGER STRENGTHENER

Benefits: Strengthens the fingers and helps prevent injuries, aches, and pains from knitting. **Props:** None

If you have a wrist or hand injury, avoid this practice.

1. On both hands at the same time, press your thumb to your pointer finger and release.
2. Press your thumb to your middle finger and release.
3. Press your thumb to your ring finger and release.
4. Press your thumb to your pinky finger and release.
5. Now go back the way you came. Press your thumb to your pinky finger and release.
6. Press your thumb to your ring finger and release.
7. Press your thumb to your middle finger and release.
8. Press your thumb to your pointer finger and release.

Repeat this sequence a total of 3 times.

(continued on next page)

(continued from previous page)

HAND ROLL
Benefits: Opens the wrists and forearms. **Props:** None

If you have a wrist or hand injury, avoid this practice.

1. Bring your hands in front of your chest and point your fingers toward the floor.
2. Gently press the backs of your hands together.
3. With the backs of your hands still touching, bring your fingertips toward your chest and up toward the ceiling. Once your fingertips are facing the ceiling, press your palms together.
4. Then bring the backs of your hands to touch again.
5. Go in the opposite direction with your fingertips pointing away from your chest.

Repeat a total of 3 times in each direction.

WRIST & FOREARM OPENER
Benefits: Warms up the forearms for knitting. **Prop:** Chair

If you have an arm or wrist injury, avoid this practice.

1. Stand in front of a chair with the seat facing you.
2. Bend your knees and place your hands shoulder distance apart on the seat of the chair. Your shoulders should be directly above your wrists.
3. Keep your palms on the seat of the chair, and slowly turn your hands away from each other until your fingers point toward you.
4. Notice if your arms are no longer straight, and gently straighten them as much as comfort allows.
5. Hold this pose while you slowly count to 10. If it feels right, gently lean from front to back or side to side to explore your limits or help you breathe through the stretching.
6. Gently release your hands, shake them out, and take a few deep breaths.

Repeat a total of 3 times.

HAND UNDER FOOT POSE VARIATION, *padahastasana*
Benefits: Creates space in the wrists and hands. **Props:** Chair, folded blanket

If you have an arm, wrist, or hand injury, avoid this practice.

1. Place a folded blanket on the seat of a chair. Stand a foot away from the chair.
2. Bend your knees and place your palms flat on the blanket-covered seat.
3. Turn your hands over so the back of each hand is on the seat and your fingers are pointing toward you.
4. Gently press the back of your hand into the chair while trying to straighten your arm.
5. If it feels comfortable, take your right knee and gently place it into the palm of your right hand. The knee will softly press into the palm, shifting the weight forward slightly as you straighten your arm, to create space in the wrist. Take 5 breaths, then release your knee and put your right foot back on the floor.
6. Lift your left knee and place it on top of your left palm. The knee will press softly into the palm, shifting the weight forward slightly as you straighten your arm, to create space in the wrist. Take 5 breaths, then release the knee and put your left foot back on the floor. Rest for a few breaths.

Repeat a total of 3 times.

> THINK OF THESE CONDITIONING EXERCISES AS AN INSURANCE POLICY AGAINST THE ACHES THAT CAN HAMPER YOUR ENJOYMENT OF KNITTING

PRACTICE

SHOULDER AND NECK OPENERS

Knitting builds up tension in our arms, neck, and shoulders by way of the tension we create in our hands. Try all of these arm, neck, and shoulder openers, then pick at least 2 or 3 to do before each knitting session.

NECK LENGTHENER

Benefits: Releases tension in the neck. **Props:** None

If you have a neck injury, avoid this practice.

1. Sitting or standing, make your spine tall.
2. Place your right hand gently over the top of the left side of your head and coax your right ear toward your right shoulder. Be careful not to place too much pressure on your head. Think of your hand as a guide.
3. Pull your shoulders back away from your ears.
4. Count 5 breaths and then gently move your right hand to the right side of your head, and slowly bring your head up without using your neck muscles.
5. Repeat on the other side.

Repeat a total of 2 times on each side.

INTERLACED FINGERS

Benefits: Lengthens the sides of the body and opens the front of the chest and upper back. **Props:** None

If you have a neck or shoulder injury, avoid this practice.

1. Interlace your fingers and face your palms away from you.
2. Bend your elbows slightly and lift your arms forward and up to try to get your biceps by your ears. If you have tight shoulders stop at a 45° angle.
3. Maintain the position of your arms and fingers while you press your shoulder blades down your back. Remember to breathe. Keep your fingers interlaced, taking care to keep both thumbs touching and both pinkies touching.
4. Extend your arms and feel your body lengthen. Notice the space created in the front of your chest. Relax your jaw and keep moving your shoulders away from your ears.
5. Count 5 slow and deep breaths. Lower your arms to your sides.
6. Rest for a few moments and then switch the interlacing of your fingers and repeat.

Repeat each interlacing direction a total of 2 times.

COW FACE ARMS, *gomukasana*

Benefits: Opens the shoulders, chest, armpits, and triceps. **Props:** Chair, strap or long straight or circular knitting needle

If you have a back, shoulder, or neck injury, avoid this posture.

1. Sit in a chair. Place the strap over your right shoulder or hold the knitting needle in your left hand.
2. Stretch your arms out to the side in a T-shape.
3. Turn your left palm to face the ceiling, and lift your arm to the ceiling so your bicep is by your ear.
4. Bend your elbow to place your left hand at the back of your head or between your shoulder blades. Grab the strap or point the knitting needle down your spine.
5. Rotate your right arm so your thumb points toward the floor. Bend your right elbow and place the back of your right hand on your lower back.
6. Slide the back of your right hand up your back until it finds the strap or the knitting needle.
7. With both hands holding the strap or needle, pull the elbows away from each other. Remember to breathe.
8. If you feel your head moving forward, open your left arm out to the side and adjust your head back, so it stays stacked on top of your body. Then hug your left arm in toward your ear.
9. Take 5 long and slow breaths and then gently release the strap or needle.
10. Shake out your arms and then repeat on the other side.

Repeat a total of 2 times on each side.

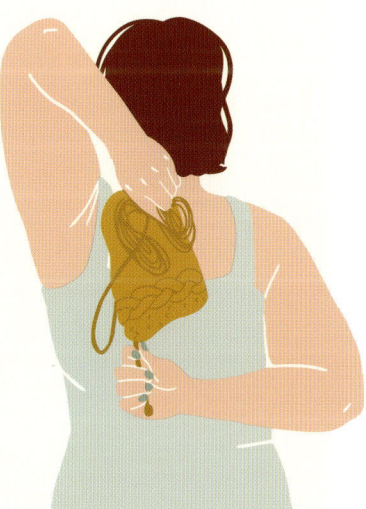

SELF-MASSAGE

Massages get the blood flowing, release tension, and work out kinks in the body. And they feel great! But most of us don't have the time or budget to get a professional massage on a regular basis. Thankfully, we can get many of the benefits when we learn how to give ourselves a self-massage.

These are my three go-to self-massages. I like to do them right after I finish knitting when my body needs a little extra love.

You need a ball and a table for these self-massages. Massage balls are great, but a tennis or lacrosse ball will do the same job. Just remember that if you're using a harder ball, like a lacrosse ball, be extra gentle, because it can bruise you if you push too hard.

HAND AND FOREARM MASSAGE

Benefits: Releases tension in the hands and forearms. **Props:** Table, chair (optional), tennis or lacrosse ball

If you have a hand, wrist, or forearm injury, avoid this practice.

1. Take the ball between the palms of your hands and roll it around. Go slowly.
2. Place the ball on the table and place your right hand down so the base of your thumb is pressing into the ball. Then, in a circular motion, slowly roll around the entire outer edge of your palm. Massage into the base of your fingers and the edge of your palm.
3. Lean into the ball with the weight of your body and try pressing on a slight angle. Remember not to apply too much pressure.
4. Take 5 to 10 deep breaths as you roll the ball while gently pressing.
5. Once you have massaged your hand fully, roll the ball up and down the front and back of your lower arm. Adjust yourself to sit or stand to make it easier.
6. Take 5 to 10 deep breaths as you roll the ball while gently pressing.

Shake out your arm and repeat on the other side.

BACK MASSAGE

Benefits: Releases tension in the back. **Props:** Wall, tennis, or lacrosse ball

If you have a back injury, avoid this practice.

1. Stand with your back against a wall. Place the ball behind your back on the right side between your spine and shoulder blade. Don't put the ball too close to your spine.
2. Press into the ball with your back.
3. Gently rock side-to-side, then up-and-down, to massage the right side of your back with the ball.
4. When you find a sweet spot, explore there. Try lifting your right arm and making slow circles to explore opening your back further.
5. Adjust so the ball gradually moves down your back without falling until it reaches your upper buttocks. Go slowly and remember to breathe.
6. Take 10 more breaths here and then remove the ball. Stand and shake out your body for a few moments.

Repeat on the other side.

FOOT MASSAGE

Benefits: Releases gripping and tension in the feet. **Props:** Wall (optional), tennis or lacrosse ball

If you have a foot injury, avoid this practice.

1. Stand tall with the ball underneath the heel of your right foot. Stand close to a wall if you want to keep one hand on it for support.
2. As slowly as you can, roll the ball from your heel to your toes. Go back and forth along the sole of your foot.
3. Take 5 to 10 deep inhales and exhales as you roll the ball.

Repeat on the other side.

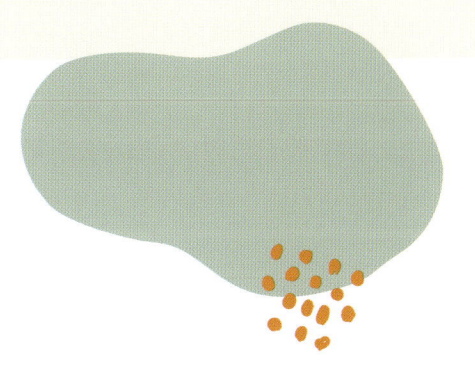

PART FOUR

joyous endeavors

In this chapter I invite you to learn through simple inhales and exhales. When we direct and guide our breath, we create space to investigate what brings us joy in yoga, knitting, and life.

SUTRA 1.34

Racchardanavdharanabhyam va pranasya.
Calm is retained by the controlled exhalation or retention of the breath.

LIFE FORCE

The direct translation of prana—the Sanskrit word for breath—is life force. We control prana through *pranayama* or breathing practices. Breathing practices reduce stress, soothe the nervous system, and change our overall attitude toward life. Yogis believe that we live longer when we train ourselves to breathe properly.

Before you try to control your breath through *pranayama* techniques, take time to watch your inhales and exhales. You can do this while knitting or at any other time that feels comfortable. Is your breathing steady or sporadic? Are you breathing into your abdomen or your chest? Do you feel the diaphragm expanding and contracting? Are you building up or releasing tension? Are you sucking in your belly rather than allowing it to expand with each inhale? I learned to suck in my belly when I was a little girl studying ballet. It wasn't until I was a young adult deepening my yoga practice that I finally learned to allow my belly to expand fully with each inhale, which is exactly what it is meant to do.

In the following Explorations, I have compiled my favorite breathing practices. If you are new to *pranayama*, start these exercises when you're not knitting. After a few days, slowly incorporate them into your stitching time. While you do them, remember to notice (without judgment!) what you're feeling in your body and mind.

This sutra explains how we can maintain our equilibrium by regulating our breath. The first step is simply to watch our inhales and exhales. Over time, as we learn to control our breathing, we find that we don't get agitated as much, even when people or situations become difficult.

THE BELLY IS DESIGNED TO EXPAND

In the early days of my yoga teacher training, I noticed how I restricted my breathing to my upper chest and didn't use the full capacity of my lungs, a combination that actually increases anxiety. To break this cycle, I started observing my breathing. I would lie down and place blankets and yoga blocks on my belly, so I could literally watch them rise and fall as I inhaled and exhaled. After doing this every day for many weeks, I started breathing properly, even when I wasn't focused on my breath. My belly started expanding fully as I breathed, even though I wasn't trying to make it happen. I realized something wonderful: The belly is designed to expand!

Benefits: Draws your attention to how you are breathing. **Props:** Blocks or books, something with a little weight to it

If you have a lung condition or can't lie flat on your back, avoid this practice.

1. Lie on your back on the floor or ground.
2. Place a block or a few books on your abdomen.
3. Take a few inhales and exhales, noticing if the items on your belly are rising and falling as you breathe.
4. Rest and breathe, watching the rise and fall for at least 10 breaths.

Repeat this practice daily for 1 week.

COUNT IN, COUNT OUT

A large nerve called the vagus nerve runs from the neck down through the diaphragm. When we extend our exhales, this nerve sends a signal to our brains to activate the parasympathetic nervous system (page 175). This, in turn, reduces our stress levels by taking us out of the sympathetic nervous system (page 178), which floods our bodies with adrenaline.

This practice is an introduction to controlling the breath by teaching us to take longer exhales than inhales. I like to do it before I start knitting or when I'm feeling a little anxious. I also encourage my young daughter to do it as she waits for the initial shock or pain of a boo-boo to wear off.

Benefits: Triggers rest-and-digest mode, reduces stress levels, and teaches us how to control the breath. **Props:** Chair or pillow

1. Sit tall in a chair or on a pillow on the floor.
2. Count slowly from 1 to 5 as you take a deep inhale.
3. Count slowly from 1 to 5 as you exhale deeply, pinning your belly button to your spine on 5.
4. Repeat this a total of 5 times and then start breathing without counting for a few minutes.
5. After a short break, count from 1 to 5 as you inhale.
6. Now count from 1 to 6 as you exhale. Try not to speed up your counting; instead, exhale for longer.
7. Repeat this a total of 5 times, extending from 6 seconds to 7, 8, 9, only on the exhales and as your comfort level allows.

RETENTION OF BREATH

There are actually 4 parts to each breath: (1) inhale; (2) space before the exhale; (3) exhale; (4) space at the end of the exhale before the new breath starts. Breath retention is the space between the inhales and exhales. When we practice retention and consciously lengthen the pauses, we rewire our breathing habits.

Benefits: Increases concentration and reduces fluctuations of the mind.
Props: Chair or pillows

If you are pregnant or have migraines or low blood pressure, avoid breath retention practices.

1. Sit tall in a chair or on a pillow on the floor.
2. Exhale completely through your mouth.
3. Seal your lips.
4. Inhale through your nostrils for a count of 5.
5. Retain your breath for a count of 5. Keep your lips sealed and jaw relaxed. Take a few regular inhales and exhales.
6. Exhale completely through your nostrils for a count of 5.
7. Hold your breath for a count of 5. Keep your lips sealed and jaw relaxed. Take a few regular inhales and exhales.

Repeat steps 2–7 a total of 5 times.

> BREATHING PRACTICES REDUCE STRESS, SOOTHE THE NERVOUS SYSTEM, AND CHANGE OUR OVERALL ATTITUDE TOWARD LIFE.

OCEAN BREATH

Ujjayi (pronounced oo-jai-ee), or Ocean Breath, is a breathing technique that constricts the back of the throat as we exhale to build heat with the air flowing out through the nose. This creates a hissing or light grunting noise that sounds like ocean waves.

Benefits: Creates warmth inside the body, improves concentration, and simultaneously energizes and relaxes the body. **Props:** Chair or pillow

If you are pregnant or have migraines or low blood pressure, avoid these practices.

1. Sit tall in a chair or on a pillow on the floor.
2. Take a deep inhale through your nose.
3. As you exhale through your mouth completely, stick out your tongue and relax your jaw.
4. Take your right hand in front of your mouth, and on your next exhale make an *Ahhhhhhh* sound, expelling breath as if you are trying to fog up your right palm.
5. Repeat the inhale and exhale to fog up your palm, but this time constrict your throat as you exhale so your *Ahhhhhhh* sounds even more like a hiss.
6. After your next inhale, keep the throat constricted and try to reproduce the fogging on your right palm, but close your mouth and exhale through your nose. The back of your throat should create a deep quiet sound similar to the sound of ocean waves, just loud enough to be audible to someone sitting next to you.

Repeat this constricted grunt of an exhale through your nose a total of 3 times. As Ocean Breath starts to feel more natural, increase your repetitions. Try practicing it while knitting, driving, or doing yoga.

ALTERNATE NOSTRIL BREATHING

Alternate Nostril Breathing, *nadi shodhana*, forces us to breathe in and out of one side of the nose at a time. This practice balances out our breathing, which naturally imbalances over the course of the day.

Benefits: Calms nerves, reduces anxiety, and boosts concentration. **Props:** Chair or pillow

If you have lung or heart concerns, asthma, or COPD, avoid this practice.

1. Sit tall in a chair or on a pillow on the floor.
2. Bring your right hand up toward your nose and close your left nostril with your right ring or middle finger.
3. Breathe in through your right nostril, but before you breathe out, close the right nostril with your right thumb and release the left nostril. Exhale through your left nostril.
4. Inhale through your left nostril, close your left nostril with your ring finger and release your thumb from your right nostril. Exhale through your right nostril.
5. Shake out your hand, breathe normally for a few moments, and then repeat a total of 10 times.

> ALTERNATE NOSTRIL BREATHING FORCES US TO BREATHE IN AND OUT OF ONE SIDE OF THE NOSE AT A TIME.

COOLING BREATH

Cooling Breath, *sitali*, is my go-to practice whenever I'm feeling a little flushed or overheated. This practice is generally avoided in the winter.

Benefits: Cools off the body and reduces fatigue. **Props:** Chair or pillow

If you have low blood pressure or a respiratory condition, avoid this breathing practice.

1. Sit tall in a chair or on a pillow on the floor.
2. Open your mouth to an O shape and stick your tongue part of the way out of your mouth.
3. If possible, curl the sides of your tongue up to form a "tube" at the tip. This is very hard for some people and very easy for others. If you can't do it, just skip this step!
4. Breathe in through the mouth or tongue, noticing how cool the breath is as you inhale.
5. Close your mouth and exhale through the nose.

BREATH OF FIRE

When I find myself in an unproductive lull—when my body stagnates and my mind starts to wander—I use Breath of Fire, *kapalbhati*, to reignite attention and energy.

Benefits: Creates warmth and energy to rejuvenate the mind and body. Strengthens the abdominal muscles, which prevents back pain. **Props:** Chair or a pillow

If you are pregnant or have low blood pressure or a respiratory condition, avoid this practice.

1. Sit tall in a chair or on a pillow on the floor.
2. Place your arms in a relaxed position on top of your thighs and pull your shoulders away from your ears.

BEE BREATH

Take Bee Breaths, *bhramari*, whenever you need a break. For example, if you notice your knitting tension is getting a little tight or you feel frustration building, put down your needles and explore this practice. You can keep your eyes open if that feels better.

Benefits: Releases frustration and anxiety so you can restore your mental flexibility. **Props:** Chair or cushion

Avoid this practice if you have a full stomach, heart condition, migraine, or any other type of headache.

1. Sitting tall in a chair or on a cushion on the floor, close your eyes.
2. Place each of your pointer fingers on the small piece of cartilage between your cheek and ear.
3. Breathe in and out through your nose. As you exhale through your nose, make a humming sound and gently press the cartilage with your fingers.

Repeat this slowly a total of 5 times.

3. Close your mouth and inhale deeply through your nose.
4. Force short breaths out of your nostrils at a vigorous, fast pace, snapping your belly button toward your spine with each exhale.
5. Your body will inhale when it needs to, so just keep forcing the breaths out in vigorous, short bursts at least 10 times.
6. Take a moment to breathe normally and come back to center.

Repeat 10 short, vigorous breaths out through the nose a total of 3 times.

OBSTACLES

Obstacles arise to remind us how dedicated we are to our journeys. The moment we say we are going to commit to a daily yoga practice, something may come up to distract us from that goal. When this happens, we have the opportunity to examine the authenticity of our desires.

If our desire isn't strong or sincere, then we easily find reasons to avoid our yoga practice. We can always find dishes or laundry to do, a book we've neglected reading for too long, or a TV series we've fallen behind on. If we follow a distraction rather than take the opportunity to practice, then maybe the distraction is what we really want. Maybe we don't want or need the benefits of our yoga practice as much as we sometimes think we do. Maybe that's worth noticing and processing—without judgment! At a minimum, paying attention helps us clarify how we make choices about our time.

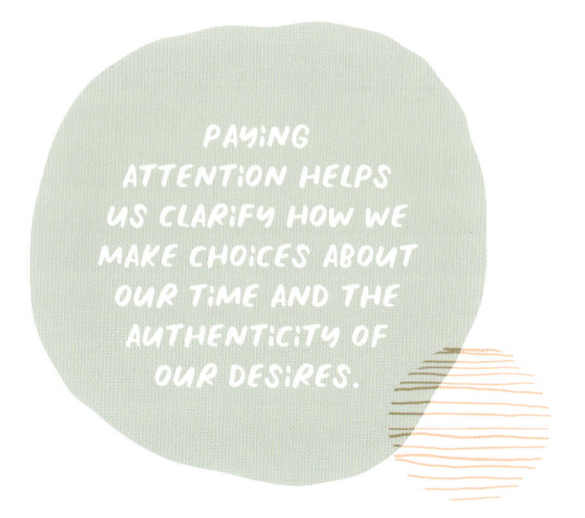

> PAYING ATTENTION HELPS US CLARIFY HOW WE MAKE CHOICES ABOUT OUR TIME AND THE AUTHENTICITY OF OUR DESIRES.

INVERSIONS

Amazingly, each part of our body feels the acceleration of almost 30 feet per second pressing against it in a single direction, downward, for our entire lives. That's gravity. Inversions are postures where the heart is above the head. When we incorporate inversions into our yoga practice, we literally reverse gravity and relieve pressure.

Child's Pose (page 42), Downward Facing Dog (page 31), Legs Up the Wall (page 144), and Bridge Pose (page 145) are all inversions. And these are poses most of us can do no matter how brittle we might feel in the moment. Bringing our hearts above our heads in any of these poses tells our bodies to relax and activates the rest-and-digest mode of our parasympathetic nervous systems.

Inversions are also a way to find that balance between strength and flexibility. We certainly gain a new perspective looking at the world upside down. Beginnings and endings blur a bit. We rest in the in-between, comfortable in that limbo, not worrying about what's next. Instead, we keep our focus on the present to maintain our balance in this inverted perspective.

When I get to the bind-off row in a knitting project, I am reminded of inversions. In both cases, I am seeking to balance strength and flexibility. And both bring me relief and a new perspective.

> **WHEN WE INCORPORATE INVERSIONS INTO OUR YOGA PRACTICE, WE LITERALLY REVERSE GRAVITY AND RELIEVE PRESSURE.**

LEGS UP THE WALL POSE

I love to do Legs Up the Wall, *viparita karani*, before I go to bed at night. It puts me in a wonderful state to transition gently into sleep.

Benefits: Reverses gravity's impact from standing and sitting all day, relieves pressure on the body, and reduces stress and anxiety. **Props:** Wall, blanket, yoga strap, bolster or pillow

If you have a heart condition or eye condition, such as glaucoma or detached retina, avoid this posture.

1. Gather your props.
2. Place the bolster or pillow a hand's distance away from the wall.
3. Sit with your back to the side of the bolster and your right hip against the wall. Your chest is perpendicular to the wall.
4. Take your hands behind you on the side of the bolster away from the wall.
5. Bend your elbows as you lean backwards, bringing your upper body down to the floor and swinging your legs up the wall.
6. Press your feet into the wall and lift your hips onto the bolster. Scoot yourself toward the wall so your bottom is off the bolster and your entire upper back is resting on the floor.
7. Extend your arms out to the sides with your palms facing up so you form a T-shape on the floor.
8. Close your eyes and rest here for at least 10 breaths and up to 5 minutes.

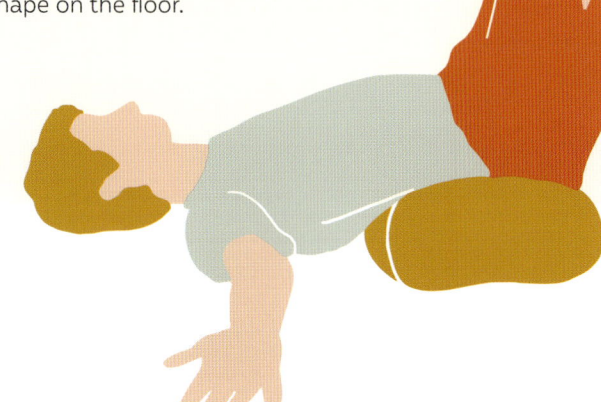

SUPPORTED BRIDGE POSE

Supported Bridge, *setu bandha sarvangasana*, is a soothing posture to help reverse the effects of rounding forward, like when we knit, text, or chop vegetables.

Benefits: Extends the spine, relieves back pain, and opens the chest.
Props: Yoga strap and 2 blocks

If you have a back injury, avoid this posture.

1. Place the strap on the floor right where you will be placing your hips.
2. Place one block within hands reach as you lie on the floor with the strap under your hips.
3. Feet flat on the floor hip distance apart.
4. Put the second block between your inner thighs.
5. Gently squeeze the block between your legs as you lift your hips and back off the floor.
6. Place the remaining block on the lowest height under your hips. Make sure the block is directly under your sacrum, closer to the upper part of your buttocks rather than your lower back.
7. Grab the strap with your hands and walk your hands as close together as you can. You'll be limited because of the location of the block, and that's okay.
8. Gripping the strap, roll your shoulders back to open the chest, and press your shoulder blades into your back.
9. Release the strap and press your palms into the floor.
10. Breathe with intention in this position for 10 breaths.

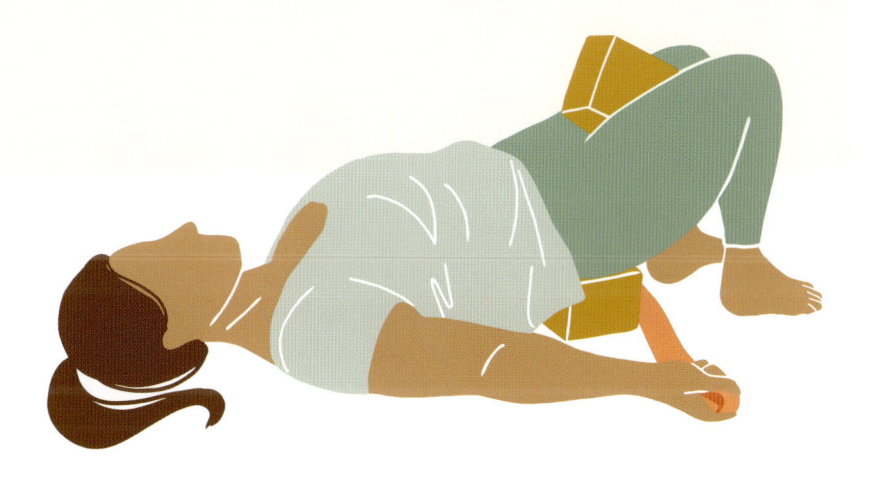

FINISHING

Once we've bound off our stitches in knitting, it's time to work our seams (if we have any), weave in ends, and block our finished objects so the stitches even out and find their final shape. We often use a tapestry needle for seaming and also to hide the ends in seams or stitches. To block, we wet the project, either by soaking it in a tub of water or spraying it with water, depending upon the fibers. Some of us add a cleanser to our water when soaking. I like to use Eucalan or Soak, neither of which needs to be rinsed out. At this point, many of us tend to rush. But finishing a knit is an especially good time to slow down so we can give our work the close attention it deserves.

We can learn something about finishing knits from yoga classes, which typically end with a restful period during which we do simple restorative poses and a mini-meditation. We don't grab our mats and race out the door. Instead, we slow down our heart rate so we can listen to each fiber of our bodies. In doing so, we give ourselves a chance to enjoy how we feel and delight in what we have accomplished. Maybe we notice what fibers feel amazing and what still needs work in the future.

When I feel myself rushing through the finishing process, I try to catch myself and change course. In the best case, I try to turn finishing into a kind of ritual. I turn on calming music and clear a space on my desk or find a comfy spot on the couch. I breathe deeply. I remember that the time I spend finishing is another opportunity for me to train my body and mind to be present. I remind myself that the fibers will absorb the energy I radiate, and I want to be kind and gentle to them. I recall the sentiment—*how we we do one thing is how we do everything* (page 122). I take myself to a calm and centered place and, in the process, I honor myself, my materials, and my work.

> WE CAN LEARN SOMETHING ABOUT FINISHING KNITS FROM YOGA CLASSES, WHICH TYPICALLY END WITH RESTORATIVE POSES AND A MINI-MEDITATION.

RESTING POSE

In many yogic traditions, the practice ends in Resting Pose, *savasana*. This is also known as Corpse Pose, or final relaxation. After all that hard work moving and stretching, we lie down with our backs flat on the floor and just breathe. This gives the body time and space to register all the benefits of the preceding movements. The yoga sinks into the fabric of the body, just like water sinks into our finished knits when we block them. At this final stage, our finished knits or our stretched bodies relax with all of the joy we've put into them.

Read through these instructions fully at least once before you take this pose, which is all about relaxation, not reading! Some days this pose is my entire home yoga practice. Other days, after I work up a good sweat, I can feel my body lengthen as I rest in *savasana*.

Benefits: Calms the central nervous system and transitions us from the end of one thing to the beginning of another. **Props:** Timer, 2 blankets, bolster or pillow, and yoga mat or rug to lie on

If you are unable to lie flat on your back, recline on an angle with multiple pillows under you for support.

1. Lie down on a yoga mat or rug.
2. Place the bolster or pillow under your knees.
3. Place one blanket under your head and neck, with the edge of the blanket rolled under your neck for support.
4. Place the other blanket on top of yourself.
5. Fiddle around with your body parts until you feel like you could rest without moving for up to 5 minutes.

6. Set your timer for 5 minutes.
7. Let your eyes close. Scan your entire body from the tips of your toes to the top of your head. Notice if you are gripping or holding tension anywhere. Release it. Shake it out if that feels right.
8. Unclench your teeth and relax your jaw. Breathe deeply in and out through your nose.
9. Bring your focus to your breath and lie still without moving for up to 5 minutes.
10. Notice when your mind wanders. Acknowledge the wandering and bring your awareness back to your breath.
11. When ready, move your head gently from side to side and wiggle your fingers and toes.
12. Stretch your arms over your head and your legs in the opposite direction. Grow your body long.
13. Bring your knees into your chest and slowly roll over to one side.
14. Thank yourself for taking 5 minutes to rest. With care, slowly bring yourself up to stand and go back to your day.

> AT THIS FINAL STAGE, OUR FINISHED KNITS OR OUR STRETCHED BODIES RELAX WITH ALL OF THE JOY WE'VE PUT INTO THEM.

JOYOUS ENDEAVORS

RECLINED BOUND ANGLE POSE

Reclined Bound Angle Pose, *supta baddha konasana*, induces rest and relaxation. It's a great alternative to *savasana* at the end of a practice or when you just need a short break. As a knitter I appreciate a gentle back-bend, because it opens up the heart center (page 174). The blankets underneath the knees give support to the joints, allowing the body to relax and open.

Benefits: Soothes abdominal discomfort and improves circulation, opens the heart center and hips. **Props:** Bolster, eye pillow, 2 blankets, and 2 yoga blocks or books

If you have severe sciatica or an injury in your knees, neck, or hips, avoid this posture.

1. Gather your props and sit down on the floor.
2. Place the bolster behind you with the short edge near your lower back so when you lie down your spine will rest along the length of the bolster.
3. Place 2 blocks or books under the bolster at the other end, where your head will rest, so the bolster rises at an angle.
4. Bend your knees and place your feet flat on the floor.
5. Take your hands to the sides of each hip, and lean back until your spine rests on the inclined bolster.
6. Bring the soles of your feet together and spread your knees apart, releasing them toward the floor.

> REST FULLY INTO THE PROPS. UNCLENCH YOUR JAW. ALLOW YOUR MUSCLES TO SOFTEN—LIKE YOUR STITCHES DO AS YOU BLOCK YOUR HANDKNITS.

7. Place a folded blanket under each knee.
8. Place the eye pillow over your eyes.
9. Lie in this position for about 5 minutes, bringing your awareness to the gentle inhales and exhales through your nose.
10. When ready, slowly roll to one side and press yourself up to standing.

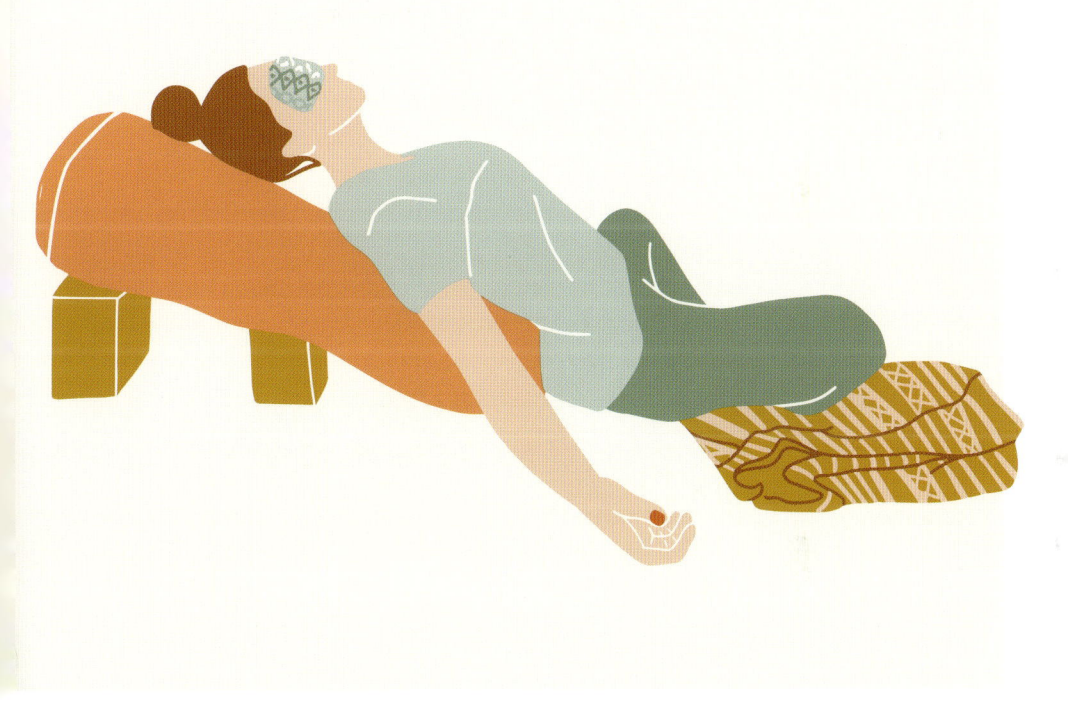

JOYOUS ENDEAVORS

BY FINDING BEAUTY IN THE IMPERFECTION IN FRONT OF US RIGHT NOW, WE CULTIVATE CONTENTMENT.

CONTENTMENT

Despite the imperfection and impermanence all of us encounter in our lives, contentment, or *santosha*, is always available to us. All we need to do is pull back the veil we drape over our minds that prevents us from seeing it. In other words, we need to get out of our own way, which is, of course, easier said than done.

By finding beauty in the imperfection in front of us right now, we cultivate *santosha*. We stop wanting or needing things to be different. We recognize that things are exactly as they should be, and everything is already okay.

When knitting, we might simply improvise to correct an error—say, work an extra decrease when our stitch count is off by one—or we might reframe an error as a design element. On our yoga mats, we accept that our Child's Pose may look different from someone else's, or that one side of the body might be a little tighter than the other. We may giggle as we wobble in Tree Pose. Or we might let out a big laugh when we just can't quiet our minds enough to follow our mantra during a meditation practice. We can make the choice to go easy on ourselves and live just a little bit lighter—because why not?

At other times, we are just anxious, restless, or emotional, and nothing we do gets us out of that funk. Here's the thing: We don't need to de-funk ourselves! We don't need to fix things! We can just sit with our feelings. We can let them have the space and time they need. And when we do, sooner or later, *santosha* comes around the corner—it was always right there!

CONTROL

Through daily repetition of practices like the ones in this book, we develop a remarkable ability to stabilize our thoughts. We learn to control our minds and ensure our thoughts serve us while letting go of everything else around us.

We appreciate better the role nonattachment (page 99) plays in our contentment. We notice what we are holding onto—what we are trying to control in our lives. When we notice the urge to arrange things in our lives according to our expectations, we let the urge pass without acting on it. We surrender more easily and, in doing so, open our ears to the voice of the universe, which always has a message for us to hear. We see that the more we attempt to control, the more muffled that message becomes.

We can notice this in our knitting too. Once we have done our gauge swatch and started a project, it's easy to get caught up in how much time we've already invested. We may notice ourselves resisting tearing out a few (or many!) rows when we find an error or realize that a different approach—maybe a change in the arrangement of the colors—might be better. We resist because we are attached.

When we feel ourselves resisting, we might benefit from asking ourselves about other situations when we have felt this way. Situations like these are a testing ground for our lives as a whole. When we learn to knit with ease and joy through nonattachment, we are able to transfer these skills to our lives as a whole—and we often do so naturally and without any extra effort.

> **THROUGH DAILY REPETITION OF PRACTICES LIKE THE ONES IN THIS BOOK, WE DEVELOP A REMARKABLE ABILITY TO STABILIZE OUR THOUGHTS.**

NO MATTER HOW LONG IT TAKES TO REALIZE A MISTAKE, ONCE WE DO, WE ALWAYS CHOOSE HOW WE REACT AND WHAT WE LEARN.

GO AHEAD AND LAUGH

Yoga and knitting are meant to be fun. No matter how seriously we take ourselves, we benefit when we are able to surrender and laugh when we make a mistake. A few years ago, I was in a yoga class working on challenging arm balances when I proved this point to myself.

Arm balances require strength, but more importantly, they require presence and focus. If the mind wanders and we lose focus on our knuckles and finger pads pressing into the floor, or forget to engage our legs, or start holding our breath, we tumble and fall. This is exactly what happened to me during that class. I got into an arm balance and held it for a couple seconds, and then I tumbled—hard! The moment I hit the ground, I burst out laughing. My classmates looked confused, but I didn't mind. I was surprised by my fall and had a childlike giddy reaction to it. Instead of feeling embarrassed, I enjoyed the reminder to keep practicing and stay present.

When knitting, we don't always realize right away that we've made a mistake. Unlike falling out of a yoga posture, it might take two or thirty rows before we notice a cable twisted in the wrong direction or a mixed-up stitch sequence. No matter how long it takes to realize the mistake, once we do, we always choose how we react and what we learn. If we choose to stay frustrated, then we're making the situation harder than it needs to be and possibly putting up an emotional barrier that will make us reluctant to try something new or challenging in the future. If we obsess about the time wasted or how long it will take to unravel back to the mistake, then we'll only make matters worse.

In these moments, even if laughing is the last thing we feel like doing, I suggest forcing a laugh, even a fake one. It's easier to act ourselves into a new way of thinking than to

154 YOGA OF YARN

think ourselves into a new way of acting. And when you fake that laugh, you may find that the frustration dissolves. If it doesn't, keep laughing! This really works, if we let it.

KNITTING WITH TEARS

Yoga is known to be a cathartic experience. It's common for yogis to experience a big emotional release while practicing. It's normal. It's encouraged. And from personal experience I can tell you that it feels great—like the reset button to end all reset buttons.

Knitting has a similar power to release pent-up emotions, as it allows us to sit with our thoughts. In my experience in classes and other social gatherings with knitters, when someone gets teary, they tend to try to hold back the waterworks. I propose that we take a lesson from the yogis and let the tears flow. Let's change the norm. Let's encourage one another to find that release through knitting. I'm not suggesting we force tears, but I am suggesting that we talk about the benefits of letting our emotions out and that we encourage each other to do so when the time comes. Few things feel better than a good cry!

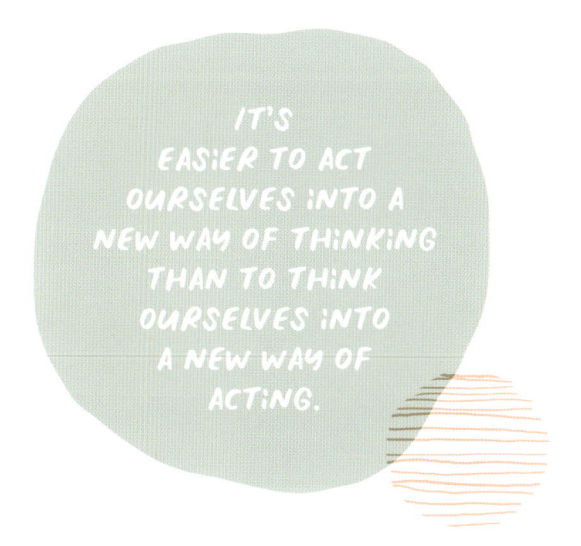

IT'S EASIER TO ACT OURSELVES INTO A NEW WAY OF THINKING THAN TO THINK OURSELVES INTO A NEW WAY OF ACTING.

SUN SALUTATIONS

Sun Salutations, or *surya namaskara* A, B, and C, are sequences of poses linked together by the breath, typically practiced at the beginning of yoga classes. This sequence of postures is designed to create warmth and prepare the body for more advanced movements. It also helps prepare us to sit in meditation for extended

SURYA K

Below and on page 158–159 you'll find two variations of *Surya K*, one that uses a chair and one that doesn't. If you're feeling restorative, try the chair version first. If you're feeling energetic, try it without the chair first.

1. Mountain Pose, *exhale*

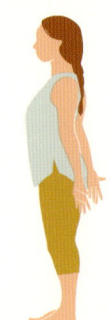

2. Upward Salute, *inhale*

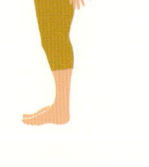

3. Forward Fold, *exhale*

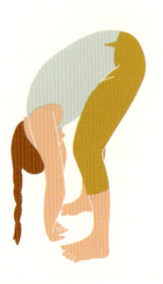

4. Half Lift, *inhale*

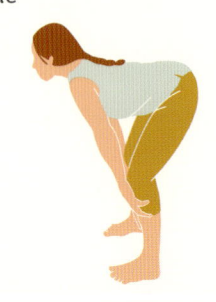

5. Table Top, *exhale*

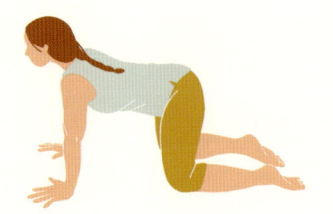

6. Cow Pose, *inhale*

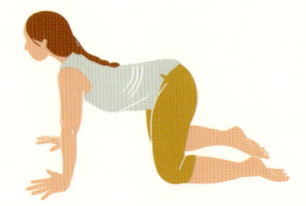

YOGA OF YARN

periods of time. Sun salutations help me knit with ease. I designed this *Surya K* version of a Sun Salutation with knitters in mind. It still builds strength, flexibility, and mental clarity, but it also emphasizes opening the chest and shoulders, which tend to round forward and tighten when knitting.

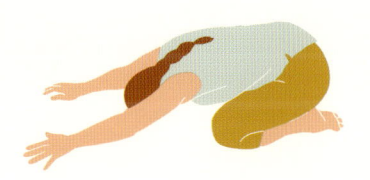

7. Child's Pose, *exhale*

8. Half Lift, *inhale*

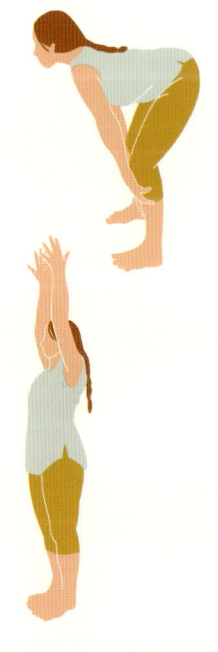

9. Forward Fold, *exhale*

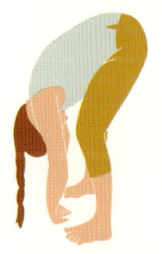

10. Upward Salute, *inhale*

11. Mountain Pose, *exhale*

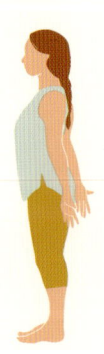

THIS SEQUENCE OF POSTURES IS DESIGNED TO CREATE WARMTH AND PREPARE THE BODY FOR MORE ADVANCED MOVEMENTS.

(continued on next page)

JOYOUS ENDEAVORS

(continued from previous page)

SURYA K WITH CHAIR

1. Mountain Pose, *inhale-exhale*

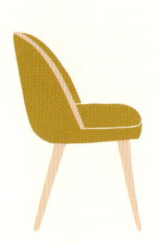

2. Upward Salute, *inhale*

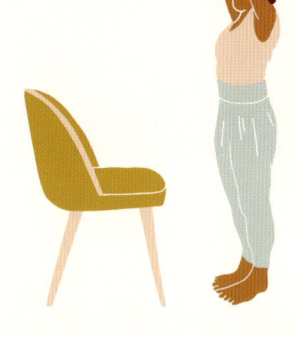

3. Forward Fold, *exhale*

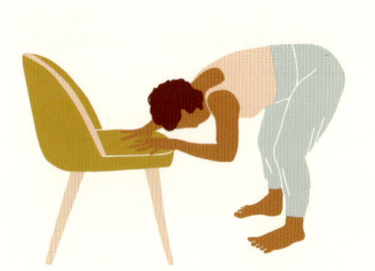

4. Half Lift, *inhale*

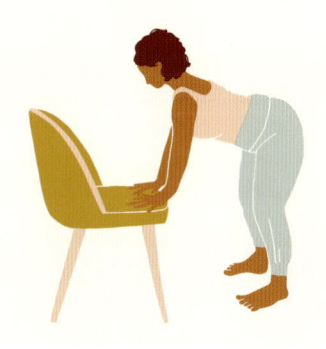

5. Plank, *exhale*

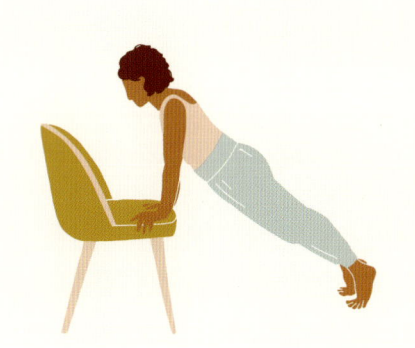

6. Up Dog, *inhale*

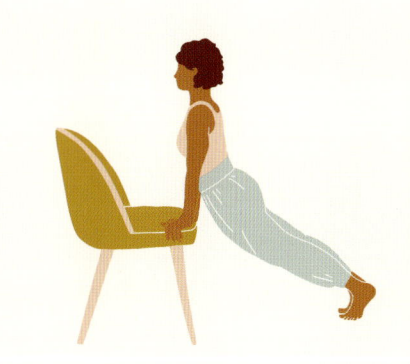

YOGA OF YARN

7. Supported Down Dog, *exhale*

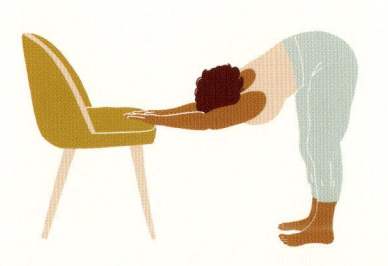

8. Half Lift, *inhale*

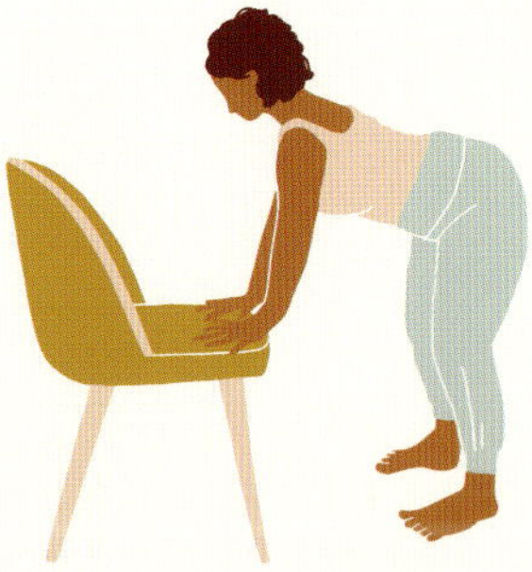

9. Forward Fold, *exhale*

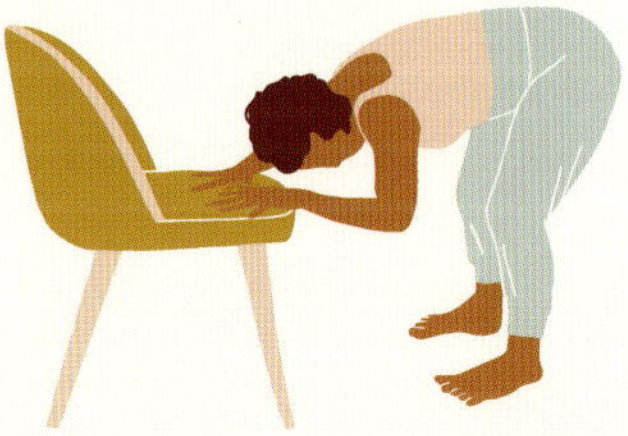

10. Upward Salute, *inhale*

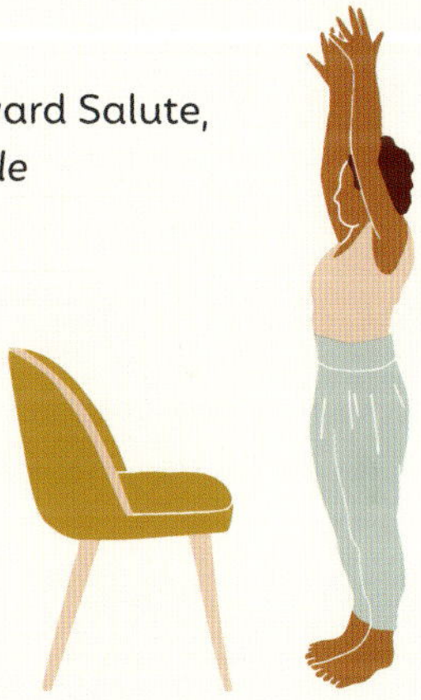

11. Mountain Pose, *exhale*

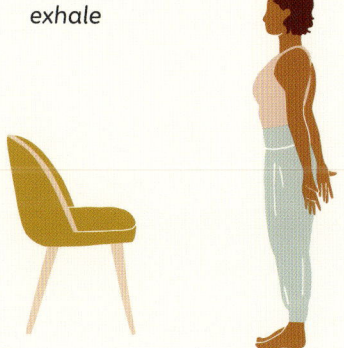

THIS VARIATION OF SURYA K IS A GENTLER ALTERNATIVE TO THE ONE ON PAGES 156–157.

JOYOUS ENDEAVORS

KNITFLIX

Once we're able to read and follow a pattern easily, or make up a pattern as we go, certain knitting sessions can start to feel as if they're mindless. We can check out mentally and still get the job done. When we start feeling this way, it's important to remember this truth: No project, even the simplest one, has to be mindless. There's always the opportunity to practice or become aware of something new. We might try out a new mantra or breathing technique. We might focus on our posture or how we are holding our yarn and knitting needles. I have found that rewiring the breath while knitting is a fresh challenge that rewards me each and every time I do it.

This isn't to say we haven't earned the right for some Knitflix. There is something so cozy and wonderful about curling up on the couch, knitting needles in hand, and watching a good movie. Or listening to an audiobook or podcast. Or having a conversation with a good friend. We get a special kind of release from doing our simple projects alongside these relaxing distractions.

As with all our practices, we benefit when we pay attention to how these comfort modes are affecting us. If we aren't mindful, a moderate twice-weekly Knitflix session can transform over a few months into a nightly Knitflix binge with aching eyes, hands, and arms. If we realize a practice isn't serving us, we don't judge. We simply correct. We act ourselves into a new way of thinking and behaving. We do this by returning to the healthy practices that work for us and rebuilding the good choices we have let slip.

> **NO PROJECT, EVEN THE SIMPLEST ONE, HAS TO BE MINDLESS. THERE'S ALWAYS THE OPPORTUNITY TO PRACTICE OR BECOME AWARE OF SOMETHING NEW.**

SLOW MO

Slow knitting is about being attentive to the knits and purls as we go: checking each row as we finish it, taking time to admire our stitches, prioritizing the process, the UFO (unfinished object) over the end result, the FO (finished object). *UFO > FO* might be the mantra of a good slow-mo knitting practice. This concept of slowness is central to yoga as well. There's no cheat code or shortcut to enlightenment. The moment we let speed win out over precision and deliberate movement, we stop doing yoga.

I still remember a day in my early twenties when I was working at my first job in New York City. I was rushing out of the subway, weighed down by three bags, when a man started chasing me and shouting, *What's the rush, lady? They won't appreciate it, so why bother?* The man had a point. And it was a point I wasn't ready to hear.

Of course, I didn't slow down. A random stranger wasn't going to make me late for work. I was running at top speed all the time during that period of my life. And I was surrounded by others moving at warp speed, too.

These days, when I notice myself going too fast, I turn to yoga. I do a home practice or head to a class where I move especially slowly and with intention, even if that means I'm not in sync with everyone else. Sometimes I'll even tell the teacher before the class begins, so he or she doesn't interrupt me. Moving with snail-paced intention and making each and every motion measured and mindful builds my strength and stability. I rely on muscles rather than momentum.

To practice moving slowly, I invite you to explore Ease as an Intention (page 9), The Belly is Designed to Expand (page 135), Body Scan (page 60), Legs Up the Wall Pose (page 144), and Walking and Knitting (page 166). Another way to slow down is to learn a new stitch or try a complicated project that is a bit outside your comfort zone. Perhaps you'll want to knit a Yoga or Meditation Mat (page 162).

> **THE MOMENT WE LET SPEED WIN OUT OVER PRECISION AND DELIBERATE MOVEMENT, WE STOP DOING YOGA.**

YOGA OR MEDITATION MAT

This asymmetrical brioche and garter stitch mat is for meditation (in the small size) or a gentle yoga practice composed of slow, deliberate movements (in the larger size). It cushions the body and adds warmth and coziness to the experience.

The larger size also works as a shawl to keep you warm as you sit in stillness.

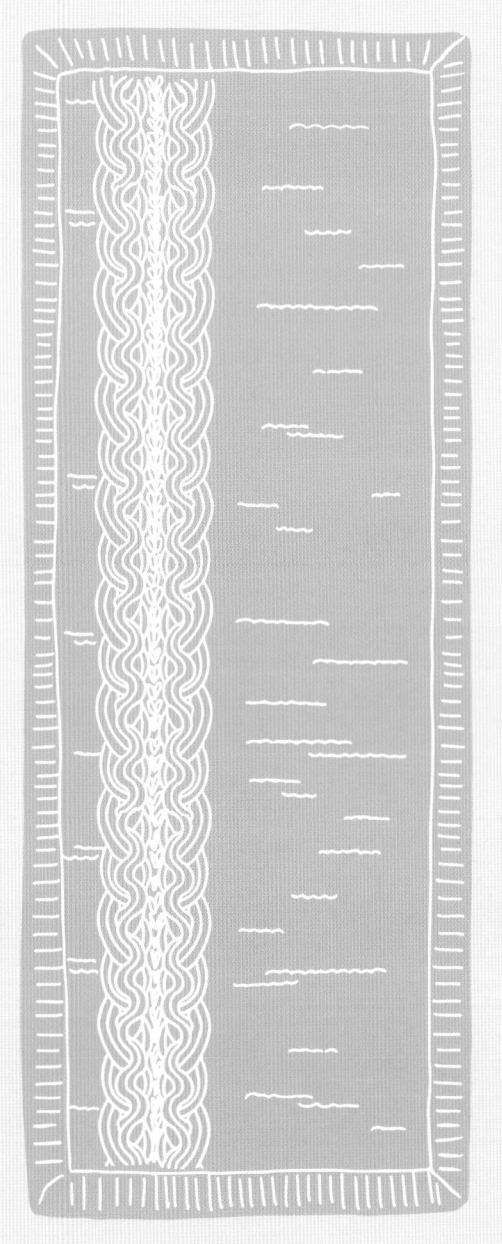

Size & Dimensions

25" [63.5 cm] wide by 29 (58)" [73.5 (147.5) cm] long

Materials

450 (900) yards [411 (823) meters] super bulky-weight yarn

Size US 10.5 (6.5 mm) 24" (60 cm) and 60" (150 cm) circular needles, or size needed to obtain gauge

4 stitch markers, including 1 unique marker for the beginning of the round

Gauge

12 stitches and 22 rows (11 Garter ridges) = 4" (10 cm) in Garter stitch, after blocking

11 stitches and 13 rows = 4" (10 cm) in Brioche Pattern, after blocking

Always use a needle size that will result in the correct gauge after blocking.

YOGA OF YARN

Mat

Cast on 62 stitches using 24" (60 cm) circular needle and Long-Tail Cast-On. Note: You may work Brioche Pattern from text or chart.

Set-Up Row 1 (RS): Knit 30, pm, work Set-Up Row 1 of Brioche pattern to last 10 stitches, pm, knit to end.

Set-Up Row 2 (WS): Knit to marker, sm, work Set-Up Row 2 of Brioche Pattern to marker, sm, knit to end.

Row 1: Knit to marker, sm, work Row 1 of Brioche Pattern to marker, sm, knit to end.

Continue working Brioche Pattern as established between the markers and Garter stitch (knit every row) on the rest of the stitches until piece measures 25.5 (54.5)" [65 (138.5) cm] from cast-on edge.

Bind off all stitches.

With RS facing, beginning at left-hand end of short edge and using longer circular needle, pick up and knit 1 stitch in each corner stitch, 1 stitch in each Garter ridge along the long edges, and 1 stitch in each cast-on or bound-off stitch along the short edges, placing a marker before each corner stitch. Join in the round and place a unique marker at the beginning of the round.

Increase Round: Kfb, *knit to 1 stitch before marker, kfb, sm, kfb; repeat from * to last stitch, kfb. (8 stitches increased)

Repeat the Increase Round until edging measures 1.75" (4.5 cm), making note of the total number of Increase Rounds worked.

Purl 1 round (Turning Round).

Decrease Round: Ssk, *knit to 2 stitches before marker, k2tog, sm, ssk; repeat from * to last 2 stitches, k2tog.

Repeat the Decrease Round until you have worked the same number of Decrease Rounds as Increase Rounds.

Fold the edging to the WS at the Turning Round. Line up the live stitches with the corresponding stitches along the pick-up ridge on the WS of the edging; you will be joining the live stitches to the pick-up ridge. *Insert the left-hand needle into a stitch along the pick-up ridge, then knit that picked-up stitch together with the first live stitch on the left-hand needle*. Repeat from * to * again, then bind off 1 stitch. Continue working in this manner until all live stitches have been bound off.

Weave in the ends and block.

(continued on next page)

(continued from previous page)

Brioche Stitch Pattern (see chart)
(panel of 22 stitches; 14-row repeat)

Set-Up Row 1 (RS): *K1, sl1yo; repeat from * to end.

Set-Up Row 2 (WS): *Brk1, sl1yo; repeat from * to end.

Row 1: Brk1, sl1yo, brkyobrk, sl1yo, brLsl dec, sl1yo, [brk1, sl1yo] 4 times, brRsl dec, sl1yo, brkyobrk, sl1yo.

Row 2: Brk1, sl1yo, K1, sl1yo, [brk1, sl1yo] 7 times, K1, sl1yo, brk1, sl1yo.

Row 3: [Brk1, sl1yo] twice, brkyobrk, sl1yo, brLsl dec, sl1yo, [brk1, sl1yo] twice, brRsl dec, sl1yo, brkyobrk, sl1yo, brk1, sl1yo.

Row 4: [Brk1, sl1yo] twice, K1, sl1yo, [brk1, sl1yo] 5 times, K1, sl1yo, [brk1, sl1yo] twice.

Row 5: [Brk1, sl1yo] 3 times, brkyobrk, sl1yo, brLsl dec, sl1yo, brRsl dec, sl1yo, brkyobrk, sl1yo, [brk1, sl1yo] twice.

Row 6: [Brk1, sl1yo] 3 times, K1, sl1yo, [brk1, sl1yo] 3 times, K1, sl1yo, [brk1, sl1yo] 3 times.

Row 7: *Brk1, sl1yo; repeat from * to end.

Row 8: *Brk1, sl1yo; repeat from * to end.

Row 9: [Brk1, sl1yo] 3 times, brRsl dec, sl1yo, brkyobrk, sl1yo, brkyobrk, sl1yo, brLsl dec, sl1yo, [brk1, sl1yo] twice.

Row 10: [Brk1, sl1yo] 4 times, K1, sl1yo, brk1, sl1yo, K1, sl1yo, [brk1, sl1yo] 4 times.

Row 11: [Brk1, sl1yo] twice, brRsl dec, sl1yo, brkyobrk, sl1yo, [brk1, sl1yo] twice, brkyobrk, sl1yo, brLsl dec, sl1yo, brk1, sl1yo.

Row 12: [Brk1, sl1yo] 3 times, K1, sl1yo, [brk1, sl1yo] 3 times, K1, sl1yo, [brk1, sl1yo] 3 times.

Row 13: Brk1, sl1yo, brRsl dec, sl1yo, brkyobrk, sl1yo, [brk1, sl1yo] 4 times, brkyobrk, sl1yo, brLsl dec, sl1yo.

Row 14: [Brk1, sl1yo] twice, K1, sl1yo, [brk1, sl1yo] 5 times, K1, sl1yo, [brk1, sl1yo] twice.

Repeat Rows 1–14 for Brioche Pattern.

Glossary

Brk1 Brioche knit 1: Knit the stitch that was slipped in the previous row together with its yarnover.

Sl1yo Slip 1, yarnover: Bring yarn under needle to the front, slip 1 stitch purlwise, then bring yarn over needle to the back before working the next stitch (this will create a yarnover when the next stitch is worked).

Brkyobrk Working into 1 stitch, brioche knit 1 (brk1), yarnover (bringing yarn under the needle first, then over the needle to the back), brioche knit 1; 2 stitches increased.

BrLsl dec Slip 1 stitch (and its yarnover) knitwise with yarn in back, brioche knit following 2 stitches together [a single stitch and a knit stitch (and its yarnover)], then pass slipped stitch (and its yarnover) over; 2 stitches decreased, slants left.

Brioche Stitch Pattern

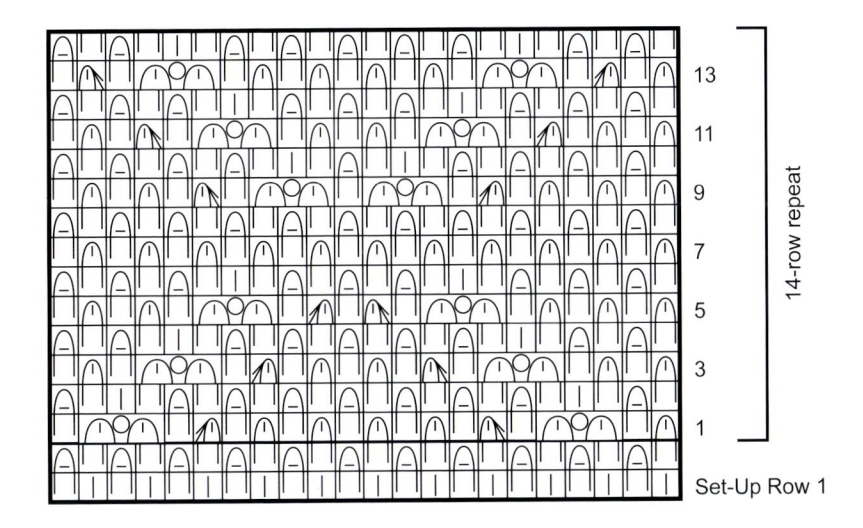

14-row repeat

Set-Up Row 1

| | K1
| | Sl1yo
| | Brk1 on RS
| | Brk1 on WS
| | BrLsl dec
| | BrRsl dec
| | Brkyobrk

BrRsl dec Slip 1 stitch (and its yarnover) knitwise, knit next stitch, pass slipped stitch (and its yarnover) over, return stitch to left-hand needle, then pass the following stitch (and its yarnover) over it; slip stitch to right-hand needle; 2 stitches decreased, slants right.

K2tog Knit 2 stitches together; 1 stitch decreased, slants right.

Kfb Knit into front and back of next stitch; 1 stitch increased.

Pm Place marker

Sm Slip marker

Ssk Slip 2 stitches one at a time knitwise to right-hand needle, slip them back to left-hand needle in their new orientation, then knit them together through back loops; 1 stitch decreased, slants left.

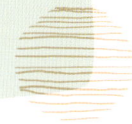

JOYOUS ENDEAVORS

WALKING AND KNITTING

In a walking meditation we focus our attention on the physical experience of stepping one foot in front of the other. With a gentle gaze on the ground, we pay close attention to the specific movements of each step, something that usually happens so naturally and automatically that we don't even think about it. We revel in slowness.

When we add knitting to the experience, we shift our perspective and see our knitting, and our bodies, in a new way.

Benefits: Boosts blood flow, reduces anxiety, and improves concentration and circulation. **Props:** Timer (optional) and a small, lightweight, easy-to-manage knitting project in a project bag you can hold on your wrist

1. Take your knitting outside to a flat clear area where you won't have to look at the ground as you walk.
2. Stand in Mountain Pose (page 14) and place your project bag around your wrist, holding your knitting in your hands.
3. Keep your chin parallel to the ground, collarbones spreading and shoulders relaxed.
4. Rest your gaze on the ground about 3 feet (1 meter) in front of you. Take your first step and let your breath and feet find a gentle rhythm together.
5. Begin knitting slowly and let your feet carry you. Walk in a wide circle, if possible.
6. Notice your posture. Avoid slouching and keep your chin parallel to the ground. Every so often, roll your shoulders back to keep them from getting tense.
7. As you walk and knit, notice the sounds around you. Do you hear the clicking of the knitting needles? Do you hear the pace of your breath? If you find yourself speeding up, slow down or come to a stop and check in with yourself.
8. Walk for at least 5 minutes. Work up to 20 minutes over time.

GRATITUDE

The practice of acknowledging what we are thankful for is one of the most important practices in our journey toward *santosha* (page 152). It costs nothing and requires no fanfare. Practicing gratitude doesn't mean we shy away from the pain and suffering in our lives. It simply puts this suffering in a different light.

When I started cancer treatments, fear and anxiety over the future gripped me constantly. Writing daily in a gratitude journal brought me back into the present. It reminded me that I couldn't control what life had in store for me, but I could control how I reacted to it. I could slow down to enjoy all the beauty that was right in front of me. I could let go and let the universe do its work.

GRATITUDE JOURNAL AND STICKY NOTES

To this day I continue to write in a gratitude journal. It's an important habit for which I make space no matter what. Sometimes, I write gratitudes on sticky notes that I place in prominent locations where I will see them often.

Benefits: Brightens our outlook and appreciation for life and all the beauty around us. **Props:** Sticky notes and/or journal, pen

1. When you wake up in the morning, write down 3 things for which you are grateful in a journal and/or on a sticky note. Do this either first thing when you roll out of bed or while you sip your first cup of tea or coffee. Be as specific as possible.

2. Place the sticky note on your bathroom mirror or refrigerator. Acknowledge what you are grateful for throughout the day and upon retiring to bed for the night.

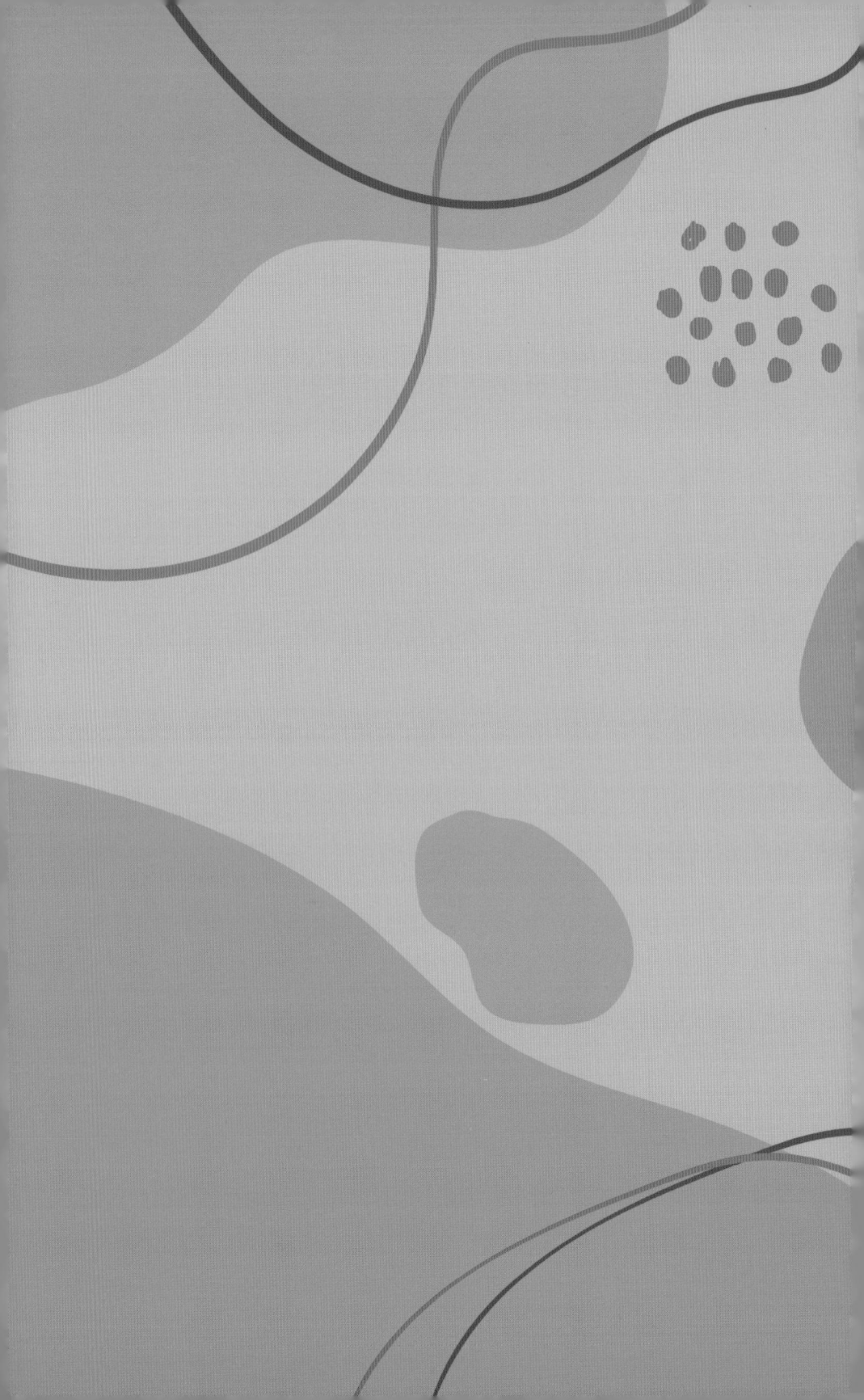

appendix

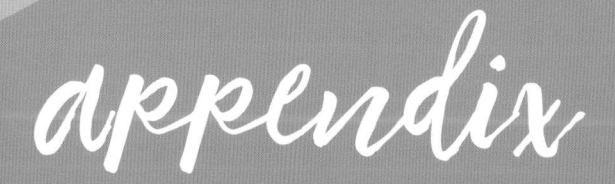

Here you will find more information to help you incorporate *Yoga of Yarn* into your daily life. There is an index of Explorations, a lexicon of yoga terminology, and a list of props, as well as some recommendations for further reading.

INDEX OF EXPLORATIONS

Yoga Postures

Easy Pose (page 12)
Posture Corrector (page 13)
Mountain Pose (page 14)
Knitter's Flow (page 19)
Knitter's Warmup (page 29)
Chakra Balancing in a Chair (page 38)
Supported Pigeon Pose (page 62)
Eye Yoga (page 85)
Eagle Arms Pose (page 88)
Seated Twist (Page 97)
Supported Fish Pose (page 113)
Hand and Wrist Prep (page 124)
Shoulder and Neck Openers (page 128)
Self-Massage (page 130)
Legs Up the Wall Pose (page 144)
Supported Bridge Pose (page 145)
Resting Pose (page 148)
Reclined Bound Angle Pose (page 150)
Surya K (page 156)

Mudras

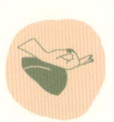

Salutation Seal (page 24)
Consciousness Seal (page 25)
Clasped Gesture (page 26)
Reverse Prayer (page 27)
Resetting with Mudras (page 102)

Meditations

Inner Energy (page 3)
Ease as an Intention (page 9)
Mantra Meditation (page 21)
Mala Cowl Meditation (page 50)
Body Scan (page 60)
Loving-Kindness Meditation (page 82)
Gratitude Journal and Sticky Notes (page 167)

Breathing Practices

The Belly is Designed to Expand (page 135)
Count In, Count Out (page 136)
Retention of Breath (page 137)
Ocean Breath (page 138)
Alternate Nostril Breathing (page 139)
Cooling Breath (page 140)
Breath of Fire (page 140)
Bee Breath (page 141)

Stitch Patterns and Practices

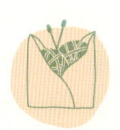

Casting On (page 16)
Brioche Mala Cowl (page 46)
Eye Pillow (page 86)
Flexible Bolster (page 112)
Yoga or Meditation Mat (page 162)

Yoga of Yarn Experiences

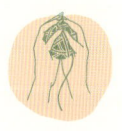

Five Principles of Sitting (page 10)
Mindful Yarn (page 23)
Knitter's Gaze (page 33)
Cultivating Intuition (page 67)
Intuitive Knitting (page 68)
Knitter's Eight-Fold Path (page 72)
Rewiring (page 79)
Needle Concentration (page 84)
What's Your Knitting and Yoga Style? (page 106)
Holding Your Needles (page 123)
Walking and Knitting (page 166)

BASIC TERMINOLOGY

If you're new to yoga or unfamiliar with its common Sanskrit nomenclature, here's a helpful guide to the basic terminology and how it relates to your yarn and knitting. Use this as needed as you explore *Yoga of Yarn*.

Term	Description
Ahimsa	One of the *yamas*, *ahimsa* means nonviolence. This includes not causing physical or emotional harm to ourselves or others. We consider where wool comes from and the local community it supports, as well as the treatment of the animals that gift us their fiber.
Aparigraha	One of the *yamas*, *aparigraha* means nonhoarding or nonattachment. A yogi does not try to grasp or cling to material things. We use our yarn, needles, and stash without hoarding, and we share with others.
Asana	Asana means seat. It is commonly used to describe the physical postures of yoga. These postures are the most common way Western culture identifies with yoga. When knitting, our asana, or posture, is usually sitting.
Asteya	One of the *yamas*, *asteya* means nonstealing, a moral principle for all humans to follow. We don't photocopy knitting patterns or otherwise avoid paying for a pattern we want to try. We don't overuse or rely on someone else's resources to their detriment because they are too nice to say no. Giving is a two-way street. We all have something to give.
Brahmacharya	One of the *yamas*, *brahmacharya* is the practice of energy conservation. It teaches us to focus our energy and spend time on what fuels us rather than what depletes us. We prioritize our projects and foster relationships that are important to us. We knit with intention—we identify why we're knitting and direct our energy to that purpose.

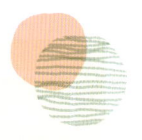

Term	Description
Chakra	Chakra means wheel and identifies the seven major energetic centers in the body. Imagine seven swirling focal points along your body's spine. Each point embodies different emotional characteristics within us. By becoming more aware of these internal workings, we learn to live in a more conscious, balanced way. We align our chakras and course-correct before we suffer for too long. When our chakras are in tune, our knits come together without frustration. When our chakras are out of whack, we can have difficulty concentrating when knitting.
Dharana	When the mind gives its undivided attention to the present moment, we experience *dharana*. *Dharana* happens when our minds and our stitches ride the same wavelength without our thoughts or bodies getting in the way.
Dhyana	*Dhyana* is part of the Eight-Fold Path (page 70), which leads to *samadhi*, the superconscious state. Often translated as meditation, *dhyana* is the training of the mind away from automatic responses toward a state of awareness.
Downward Facing Dog	Downward Facing Dog is one of the most common yoga poses. The body takes an inverted V shape with the hands and feet on the floor and hips in the air. Modified versions of this pose use a chair or wall for support (page 31). Downward Facing Dog opens up the back of the body, which gets tight from sitting and knitting.
Drishti	*Drishti* means gaze. Choosing a focal point develops concentration. While knitting, our gaze is on our needles and yarn, allowing us to become absorbed in the present, which in turn guides us toward meditation.

(continued on next page)

(continued from previous page)

Term	Description
Flow	Flow yoga is a *Vinyasa* style where movements are performed in a graceful and linked manner. The breath mediates the transition from one posture to the next in a rhythmic fashion. When we create stitches, we are in a knitting flow.
Heart Center	The heart center is the center of the chest. The instruction to lift the heart center encourages us to lift and open the chest. Lifting the heart center while knitting prevents the shoulders and back from rounding forward, which closes off the chest, causes neck and back pain, and drains energy.
Isvara pranidhana	One of the *niyamas*, *isvara pranidhana* means surrender. When we allow ourselves to believe in a power greater than ourselves and look beyond ourselves, we start to experience change from within. A deep peace emerges when we realize we are here to serve that greater power and that we can trust the universe to support us. We cast on our next project with peace and faith that what should happen will happen, whatever that may be.
Mantra	A mantra is a word or phrase repeated over and over again. For example, while knitting, the verbal repetition of the sequence *knit 1, purl 1* is a mantra.
Moving Meditation	Moving meditations use some kind of rhythmic body movement to create a single-pointed focus that quiets the mind. I find that moving meditations are the best entry points for people new to or skeptical of meditation. Knitting can be a moving meditation.

Term	Description
Mudra	Mudra means seal or gesture, and mudras are often practiced using the hands and fingers. These hand gestures improve concentration in meditation and yoga postures. We consider how we hold our knitting needles. No matter our specific style of knitting—Continental, English, Portuguese—the connection of the yarn, needles, and hands help us channel our energy.
Namaste	Namaste means "the light within me honors the light within you." Or we might say, the knitter within me sees the knitter within you. We are not so different; in fact, the more space we create to see one another, the more we realize our fundamental sameness.
Niyama	The *niyamas* are behaviors or habits related to how we care for ourselves. There are five *niyamas*: *shaucha* (purity), *santosha* (contentment), *tapas* (self-discipline to accept and not cause pain), *svadhyaya* (study of ourselves and spirituality), and *isvara pranidhana* (surrender to the greater power). These five *niyamas* relate to our own personal experiences while knitting.
Om (or aum)	Om is the sound of the universe. Believed to be the vibration of the fabric of the universe, it is a common mantra. While knitting garter-stitch, *om* is a simple mantra we can repeat to keep the mind in the present.
Parasympathetic Nervous System	The parasympathetic nervous system, also known as the rest-and-digest system, allows us to conserve energy, slow our heart rate, and ease digestion. It's the part of the nervous system that takes over after eating, when our bodies ask us to take it easy. Some of our other basic functions like crying, pooping, peeing, salivating, and sexual stimulation are also managed by the parasympathetic nervous system. When we knit, meditate, or practice yoga, we activate the parasympathetic nervous system.

(continued on next page)

BASIC TERMINOLOGY

(continued from previous page)

Term	Description
Sacrum	The sacrum is a triangular-shaped bone between the hip bones and below the last lumbar vertebra (L5) of the lower back. This small bone compresses when we sit for extended periods of time. As knitters, we try to create space to reduce the chance of lumbar pain. Good techniques to do this include Supported Child's Pose (page 42), and Supported Bridge Pose (page 145).
Samadhi	*Samadhi* means intense concentration, a hyper-conscious state achieved through meditation. This is often considered the state of enlightenment reached through fully absorbed contemplation. We may sometimes experience a high level of intense concentration while knitting something that feels complex to us, where time seems to stop and we become one with our stitches. This is *samadhi*.
Sanskrit	Sanskrit is a classical language of India. Because the Yoga Sutras (page 179) were written in Sanskrit, and yoga originates from India, we use Sanskrit terms to honor the heritage of yoga. Just as knitting terms like tink, frog, ssk, and k2p take on special meanings within our craft, the old language of Sanskrit carries a potency that the English translations do not fully capture.
Santosha	One of the *niyamas*, *santosha* translates to contentment. Contentment, or being satisfied with what we have, reminds us to focus on the project in our hands. It also expresses the concept of loving and accepting imperfections, as nothing in life is perfect or permanent. Because the world is ever-changing, we find our peace within.

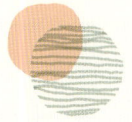

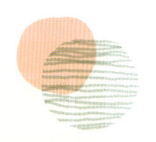

Term	Description
Satya	*Satya* means truth, or not lying. It asks us to live in a way that honors our highest truth. When we practice *satya*, we are honest with ourselves and others, and we refrain from judgment. We act and speak with intention. We take a breath before we speak and ask ourselves if what we are about to say will serve another person or if we are seeking to prove or gain something. This ensures our truth supports a selfless purpose before we bring it into the world.
Shaucha	One of the *niyamas*, *shaucha* means cleanliness and asks us to take care of our bodies and minds. We take showers not only to clean our bodies, but also to clear our minds and reset our thought patterns. We keep our yarn, needles, and supplies in good shape so they will serve their purpose in supporting our knitting practice for a long time to come. These are steps toward *shaucha*.
Savasana	*Savasana* is the term for Final Rest, or Corpse Pose. This is the final pose in a yoga class, but we can take this pose anytime. We simply lie on our backs and stretch out our arms and legs on the floor. *Savasana* is a nice way to rest after knitting and before going back to our day—or if a particularly tricky brioche increase has us frustrated and we just need a break!
Shanti	*Shanti* means peace. Commonly, *om shanti* is chanted at the close of a yoga class to seal the practice and invoke peace and calm. While knitting a challenging purl 5 together, we can try repeating *om shanti* to hold tranquility.
Sun Salutations	Sun salutations are particular sequences of postures that warm up the body for more challenging movements. *Surya* A, B, and C are common patterns. I have created what I call *Surya* K for knitters (page 156).

(continued on next page)

(continued from previous page)

Term	Description
Sympathetic Nervous System	The sympathetic nervous system, also referred to as the fight-or-flight response, is the part of the body's nervous system that responds to stressful situations. If you find yourself in a stressful situation, your heart rate may increase, raising hormone levels, making the body alert. It is the body's natural way of protecting itself in a dangerous situation. It's a state of being we aren't meant to be in for long. Practices like knitting and yoga help us stay calm and ensure we only activate our fight-or-flight response when we really need it.
Svadhyaya	One of the *niyamas*, *svadhyaya* is the examination of our self and spirituality, often through the study of spiritual books. It emphasizes our commitment to growth. Reading knitting patterns, magazines, and essays is a great way to promote our growth and knowledge of ourselves as knitters.
Tapas	One of the *niyamas*, *tapas* is self-discipline. The main way we practice *tapas* is through dedication to our craft through continuous practice. Showing up and doing the work requires constant repetition. We are better able to do this when we meditate and quiet our minds. Even when our stitches fall off our interchangeable needles, or a sweater felts in the wash, we keep going.
Ujjayi	*Ujjayi* means victorious breath or ocean breath. By engaging the lungs and mind in *ujjayi*, we create warmth within the body. We enhance concentration on the task at hand, whether that be a yoga posture or a tricky lace pattern.

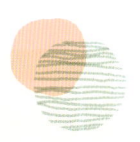

Term	Description
Vinyasa	*Vinyasa* means to place in a special way. It is the common term for flow yoga where breath links a sequence of movements. I like to think of brioche knitting as a *Vinyasa*. We place the yarn in a special way to create a plush, squishy fabric. There is a natural flow and order to the knitting sequence, and brioche goes a lot more smoothly when we breathe through it!
Yama	The *yamas* are ethical considerations concerning our relationships with others and ourselves. We consider these five *yamas* in our interactions with fellow knitters: *ahimsa* (nonviolence), *satya* (truthfulness), *asteya* (nonstealing), *brahmacharya* (energy conservation), and *aparigraha* (nonattachment).
Yoga Sutras of Patanjali	The *Yoga Sutras of Patanjali* are threads of wisdom explaining the spiritual and physical aspects of yoga. Sutra means thread, and can refer to aphorisms or a collection of aphorisms in the form of a manual. The *Yoga Sutras* are a guide to self-study and self-understanding and can be referenced by knitters and yogis alike for deeper knowledge of the self.
Yogi	Yogi is the term for a practitioner of yoga. Whether we have taken only one yoga class or we have been practicing for ten years, we are yogis. Similarly, whether we have knit our first or our thousandth scarf, we are knitters. We choose how to identify; no one else can make that decision for us.

BASIC PROPS

Most of the practices in this book can be done without any props, except perhaps a chair. But, in case you are curious, here is a guide to props that can support your yoga and knitting practices.

Prop	Description
Bolster	A large round or rectangular pillow used during Restorative yoga postures as a support to lift the body. Smaller bolsters are used for breathing practices and for support while sitting and meditating.
Chair	A seat with a back and four legs that can be used for so much more than sitting!
Meditation Cushion	A meditation cushion, or zafu, is a round or curved cushion to sit on while meditating. It keeps the hips higher than the knees and prevents gripping in the lower body.
Massage Ball, Tennis Ball, or Lacrosse Ball	A small ball for self-massage, to release fascia and muscle tightness.

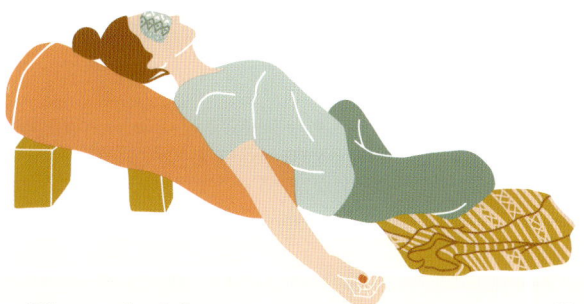

What to look for

A large supportive round bolster measures about 22" (56 cm) long and 10" (25 cm) - 12" (30 cm) in diameter. Use under your belly and chest during Child's Pose to release stress on your knees and create more space for your body to relax.

A simple folding chair will do, as will almost any other chair you have in your home. Just make sure it's sturdy, has a straight back, and doesn't have wheels or too much cushioning.

Look for a soft cushion filled with buckwheat hulls. The buckwheat creates a soft but sturdy seat that will endure daily use over time.

Massage balls are a happy medium between the firmness of the lacrosse ball and the softness of the tennis ball. Lacrosse balls are hard, so if you are new to self-massage, start with a tennis ball. Be careful, as you can bruise yourself if you press too hard. Take it easy and progress slowly.

How knitters can use

Sit on a larger bolster while knitting or place a smaller one behind your back for support.

Sit on it while knitting, of course. To prevent sinking into the lower back, place a small blanket or towel underneath the hips. During knitting breaks, use the chair as a prop for stretching.

Place the meditation cushion on the floor and sit on it while knitting.

Place the ball between your back and the back of a chair to massage your back as you knit. Hold the ball in your hand and massage it against your opposite forearm to release tension during knitting breaks.

(continued on next page)

BASIC PROPS

(continued from previous page)

Prop	Description
Timer	A device to activate or determine a preset amount of time.
Yoga Blocks	Small brick-shaped blocks used to adjust the distance between your body and the floor while practicing yoga postures.
Yoga Mat	A rectangular piece of material laid on the floor to offer a light cushion while practicing yoga postures.
Yoga Strap	A long skinny strip of nonstretchy fabric that makes it easier to stretch and reach parts of the body in certain yoga postures.

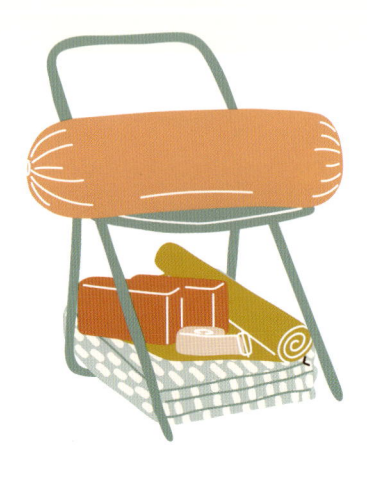

What to look for

Many mobile phones have a timer app built in.

Look for blocks made out of cork or wood. Foam blocks are mushy, topple over easily, and can cause pain in the wrists.

Look for one that is sticky to avoid slipping. If you have sensitive knees, grab a mat with extra cushioning. If you prefer a sturdier surface, pick a thinner mat and use a yoga blanket for support under the knees. Woven mats are also pleasant for slow-moving practices.

Yoga straps come in 6' (183 cm), 8' (244 cm), and 10' (305 cm) sizes. Some straps have D-rings to connect into a loop.

How knitters can use

Set a timer for 20–30 minutes to remind yourself to take a break and try an Exploration.

Place the blocks on the floor and sit on them to lift your hips above your knees. Or place two blocks on the floor under your feet while knitting in a chair.

Lay a mat underneath yourself while you knit on the floor to create warmth. Try a *Restorative* yoga pose between rows.

Use to correct your posture and keep your chest open while knitting or to keep your lower back from rounding while seated.

FURTHER READING

This book is just a stepping-stone into the world of yoga, meditation, and breathing practices. If you want to dive deeper, explore these transformative texts.

Carroll, Cain, and Carroll, Revital.
Mudras of India: A Comprehensive Guide to the Hand Gestures of Yoga and Indian Dance. Singing Dragon, 2013.

Chödrön, Pema.
Comfortable with Uncertainty: 108 Teachings on Cultivating Fearlessness and Compassion. Shambala, 2003.

Cope, Stephen.
Yoga and the Quest for the True Self. Bantam Books, 1999.

Dass, Ram.
Be Here Now. Harmony, 1978.

Dass, Ram.
Paths to God: Living the Bhagavad Gita. Three Rivers Press, 2004.

Desikachar, T. K. V.
The Heart of Yoga: Developing a Personal Practice. Inner Traditions International, 1999.

Devi, Nischala Joy.
The Secret Power of Yoga: A Woman's Guide to the Heart and Spirit of the Yoga Sutras. Three Rivers Press, 2007.

Easwaran, Eknath.
Essence of the Upanishads: A Key to Indian Spirituality. Nilgiri Press, 2009.

Farhi, Donna.
Yoga Mind, Body & Spirit: A Return to Wholeness. Holt Paperbacks, 2000.

Feuerstein, Georg.
The Deeper Dimension of Yoga: Theory and Practice. Shambala, 2003.

Iyengar, B. K. S.
Light on Life: The Yoga Journey to Wholeness, Inner Peace, and Ultimate Freedom. Rodale Books, 2006.

Iyengar, B. K. S.
Light on Prāṇāyāma: The Yogic Art of Breathing. The Crossroad Publishing Company, 1918.

Iyengar, B. K. S.
Light on Yoga: The Bible of Modern Yoga—Its Philosophy and Practice—by the World's Foremost Teacher. Schocken Books, 1979.

Judith, Anodea.
Eastern Body, Western Mind: Psychology and the Chakra System as a Path to the Self. Celestial Arts, 2004.

Judith, Anodea.
Wheels of Life: A User's Guide to the Chakra System. Llewellyn Worldwide, 1987.

Kabat-Zinn, Jon.
Coming to Our Senses: Healing Ourselves and the World Through Mindfulness. Hyperion, 2005.

Kabat-Zinn, Jon.
Wherever You Go There You Are: Mindfulness Meditation in Everyday Life. Hyperion, 1994.

Lokos, Allan.
Patience: The Art of Peaceful Living. Penguin Group, 2012.

Lokos, Allan.
Pocket Peace: Effective Practices for Enlightened Living. Penguin, 2010.

McCall, Timothy.
Yoga as Medicine: The Yogic Prescription for Health and Healing. Bantam Books, 2007.

Mitchell, Stephen.
Bhagavad Gita: A New Translation. Three Rivers Press, 2000.

Mohan, A. G., and Mohan, Indra.
Yoga Therapy: A Guide to the Therapeutic use of Yoga and Ayurveda for Health and Fitness. Shambala, 2004.

Roach, Geshe Michael.
The Diamond Cutter: The Buddha on Managing Your Business and Your Life. Doubleday, 1952.

Satchidananda, Swami.
The Yoga Sutras of Patanjali. Integral Yoga Publications, 1990.

Yogananada, Paramhansa.
Autobiography of a Yogi. Crystal Clarity Publishers, 1946.

FURTHER READING

ACKNOWLEDGMENTS

With the utmost gratitude, I shared the joy and journey of creating this book with a few generous humans. I acknowledge and thank each of them deeply for their time, guidance, and unyielding support. Kate Madden, my partner and co-conspirator at Ragline Knits, was endlessly supportive and served as a sounding board for the book's many concepts and practices. Melanie Falick, an author and inspiration to me for years before meeting her, helped structure and organize all of the concepts and practices and make them accessible to a broader audience. My closest friend and fellow yogi Erica Saccente, a contemplative psychiatric nurse practitioner, helped me grapple with the philosophies that ground the teachings in the book. Laura McFadden, a friend and Yoga + Yarn Retreat regular, used her stellar graphic design skills to visually organize and elevate my ideas. Aly Miller brought clarity and whimsy to the text with her illustrations of yogis and knitted objects. The project received a fresh perspective from Mary Neal Meador, who provided detailed support while copy editing and proofreading. Finally, my husband, Tom Scaramellino, provided endless moral support through all of the ups and downs of bringing *Yoga of Yarn* to life.

IN CLOSING

Thank you for being with me on this journey. I am endlessly grateful for you, dear reader, for taking precious time out of your day to put this guide to work for you. I love to share what I have learned, and I hope you have found something to take with you. May you be healthy, knit often, move with grace, and love freely. *Namaste.*